GLUTEN-FREE

TIPS AND TRICKS

FOR VEGANS

ALL THE FAB FOOD YOU THOUGHT YOU COULDN'T EAT

Jo Stepaniak, MSEd

Book Publishing Company
SUMMERTOWN, TENNESSEE

Library of Congress Cataloging-in-Publication Data

Names: Stepaniak, Joanne, author.
Title: Gluten-free and vegan : what to eat when you can't eat gluten / Jo
  Stepaniak, MSEd.
Description: Summertown, Tennessee : Book Publishing Company, [2016] |
  Includes bibliographical references and index.
Identifiers: LCCN 2015036705| ISBN 9781570673313 (pbk. : alk. paper) | ISBN
  9781570678615 (e-book)
Subjects: LCSH: Gluten-free diet. | Veganism. | Gluten-free diet--Recipes. |
  Vegan cooking.
Classification: LCC RM237.86 S745 2016 | DDC 641.5/636--dc23
LC record available athttp://lccn.loc.gov/2015036705

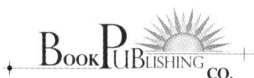

BookPublishing co.

We chose to print this title on sustainably harvested paper stock certified by The
Forest Stewardship Council, an independent auditor of responsible forestry practices.
For more information, visit https://us.fsc.org.

© 2016 Jo Stepaniak

FSC
www.fsc.org

MIX

Paper from
responsible sources

FSC® C000000

Cover Photos: Alan Roettinger
Cover and interior design: John Wincek
Stock photography: 123 RF

Printed in the United States of America

Book Publishing Company
PO Box 99
Summertown, TN 38483
888-260-8458
bookpubco.com

ISBN: 978-1-57067-331-3

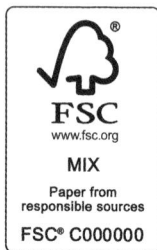

Disclaimer: The information in this book is
presented for educational purposes only.
It isn't intended to be a substitute for the
medical advice of a physician, dietitian, or
other health care professional.

21 20 19 18 17 16   1 2 3 4 5 6 7 8 9

CONTENTS

LET'S GET COOKING!

INTRODUCTION

G oing gluten-free is among the hottest new dietary crazes of the twenty-first century, and vegans haven't been immune to it. The trend has resulted in a resounding response from food manufacturers eager to ride the latest culinary wave and reap the financial rewards of catering to a rapidly growing segment of fashion-forward foodies.

Although for some vegans avoiding gluten is a choice—a way to participate in the trendiest diet du jour—for many others it's a vital necessity, and for some people it's even a matter of life and death. While there are indeed health benefits for people who are forced to abandon gluten because of a true intolerance to it, omitting something this ubiquitous can be overwhelming and life changing. So for everyone else, it's crucial to know that giving up gluten can mean unnecessarily cutting out important sources of nutrients.

Even though a gluten-free diet is recommended by some health practitioners for certain conditions unrelated to overt gluten sensitivity, such as autism spectrum disorders, please be aware that ditching gluten isn't a fast track to weight loss or a cure for chronic diseases, such as diabetes and high blood pressure. It's always a good idea to check with your health care provider before embarking on any diet that would entail eliminating broad categories of foods.

This is particularly significant for vegans, especially newbies. That's because moving to a gluten-free diet entails not only adopting an entirely new way of eating but also learning which additional foods, ingredients, and situations must be avoided, beyond those that aren't suitable for vegans in general. It can be scary and overwhelming.

This book provides an overview of the reasons many people have given gluten the heave-ho. It also covers the basics of celiac disease and gluten intolerance, how vegans can make the leap to a gluten-free diet, what to look out for when shopping, and how to stay safe when dining out. In addition, you'll find tips on gluten-free vegan cooking and baking, along with a slew of easy, delicious recipes to get you joyfully started on the right track . . . and stay there.

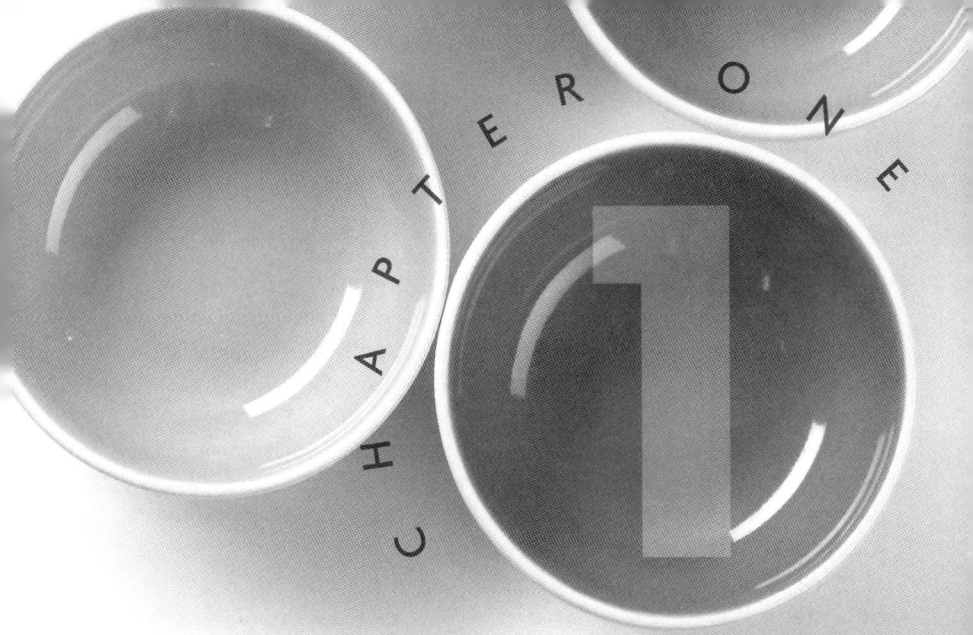

CHAPTER ONE

Celiac Disease and Gluten Sensitivity

Celiac Disease

Approximately one in 133 Americans suffers from celiac disease, also known as coeliac disease, celiac sprue, nontropical sprue, and gluten-sensitive enteropathy. An estimated eighteen million Americans have a sensitivity to gluten, and three million Americans have celiac disease. Unfortunately, most of these people live unaware of the disease and remain undiagnosed. In fact, it has been estimated that 95 percent of people with celiac disease don't know they have it.

Gluten is one of the primary proteins found in wheat and the various strains related to wheat, such as einkorn, emmer, Kamut, triticale (a grain that's a cross between wheat and rye), and spelt. It's also prevalent in barley and rye. Gluten gives bread its elasticity and helps baked goods retain their shape. For people with celiac disease, eating a food or even crumbs of food containing gluten leads to a wide array of adverse symptoms ranging from general discomfort to malnutrition and, in children, failure to grow. Wheat, barley, and rye are the primary but not only grains that people with celiac disease must avoid. They must also avoid all foods that contain gluten naturally and any processed foods to which gluten has been added (see pages 9–10).

What Is Celiac Disease?

Celiac disease is an autoimmune disorder that can occur in genetically predisposed individuals. For people with celiac disease, the ingestion of gluten mounts an immune response in the body that attacks the small intestine. These attacks lead to damage of the villi, the small fingerlike projections that line the small intestine and that promote nutrient absorption. When this structural damage occurs, nutrients can't be absorbed properly into the body, and this typically leads to malnutrition and related complications.

Celiac disease can develop at any age, but it will only occur after a person begins ingesting foods or medicines that contain gluten. If celiac disease remains untreated, it can potentially lead to or may be associated with additional serious health problems, including anemia, dermatitis herpetiformis (a skin manifestation of celiac disease that results in itchy bumps or blisters that resemble herpes lesions), early-onset osteoporosis or osteopenia, epilepsy, infertility, intestinal lymphomas and other gastrointestinal cancers, migraine headaches, miscarriage, multiple sclerosis, other autoimmune disorders, pancreatic insufficiency, type I diabetes, and vitamin and mineral deficiencies.

Symptoms and Consequences

People diagnosed with celiac disease will experience various combinations of symptoms and levels of severity. Many of these symptoms tend to mimic those of other illnesses, such as Crohn's disease, diverticulitis, irritable bowel syndrome, and ulcerative colitis. Consequently, it's not surprising to learn that people often live with the disease for a long time before a correct diagnosis is made.

Because the disease originates in the small intestine, which is where we absorb much-needed nutrients from food, celiac disease can wreak havoc on our health. Beyond nutritional deficiencies and digestive issues, such as abdominal pain, bloating, and diarrhea, a wide range of additional symptoms could result. A few of the possible consequences of untreated celiac disease include the following: anxiety, bone and joint pain, depression, fatigue, hair loss, infertility, migraine headaches, muscle wasting, neurological manifestations, skin rashes, and unintentional weight loss.

Even though celiac disease has its origins in the small intestine, it tends to manifest in systems and organs throughout the body. This is because our intestines are not only vital for our absorption of nutrients but are also the main center of immune activity in the body. At first glance it might not be obvious why symptoms such as anxiety and migraine headaches would be caused by gluten intolerance. But once we understand the role our small intestine plays in both our nutritional status and the function of the immune system, we can see how damage to that part of the body can lead to a host of other problems.

Remarkably, a small number of people with confirmed celiac disease present mild symptoms or none at all. This is what is known as "silent" celiac disease. But even if few symptoms are manifested, the consequences of consuming gluten are the same as for anyone else with celiac disease.

Diagnosis

Blood tests are commonly used to diagnose celiac disease, even though they are not 100 percent accurate. The gold standard and most accurate way to diagnose celiac disease is by an endoscopic biopsy. A diagnosis of celiac disease should not be made without a biopsy because the actual cause of symptoms may be due to a different disorder. Whether testing is done via blood work, a biopsy, or both, it's essential to maintain a gluten-containing diet before any tests are done in order for the test results to be accurate.

Treatment

There is no known cure for celiac disease. Complete and permanent avoidance of gluten is the only treatment that will avert symptoms and heal the intestine.

Gluten Sensitivity without Celiac Disease

Not all people who react negatively to gluten actually have celiac disease, even though the symptoms of gluten sensitivity may be similar to those of celiac disease. People who have gluten sensitivity certainly experience symptoms in response to eating gluten, but they don't undergo the intestinal damage that occurs with celiac disease. In addition, they will test negative for celiac disease antibodies.

You don't need a confirmed diagnosis of celiac disease to benefit from a gluten-free diet. Even if a biopsy of the intestine is normal and blood tests are negative, it's possible that your body has become sensitized to gluten in different ways that are not detected by these indicators and for which there are currently no medical tests. Some researchers postulate that gluten-sensitive people who test negative for celiac disease will eventually contract the disease. When that happens, the disorder is referred to as "latent celiac disease."

The only way to know for sure whether you are sensitive to gluten is to perform an elimination diet, during which gluten is completely avoided. This is then followed by a food challenge, which is a period when gluten is reintroduced to the diet.

Bear in mind that there's a difference between gluten sensitivity and wheat sensitivity, and while the diet therapy for each overlaps, it's an important distinction. If you test negative for celiac disease but find that you are extremely sensitive to gluten, follow the dietary advice given for celiac disease. However, some gluten-sensitive people appear to be able to tolerate small amounts of gluten or only certain types of gluten-containing foods. For example, you may be able to tolerate sprouted grain bread, true sourdough bread, or spelt sourdough bread but not regular wheat bread. The only way to know with certainty is to follow a controlled test diet and carefully track your symptoms.

Reclaiming Health with Celiac Disease

The following three-pronged approach is the best way for people with celiac disease to reclaim excellent health:

1. Avoid gluten.
2. Replenish nutrients.
3. Heal damaged intestines.

Avoid Gluten

The first and most important step to healing after being diagnosed with celiac disease is to avoid gluten in all its forms, including even microscopic amounts. People with celiac disease must follow a strict gluten-free diet and must remain on the diet for the remainder of their lives.

Nevertheless, for people with celiac disease a gluten-free diet is by no means a cure-all. In some very severe cases, a gluten-free diet alone can't halt the symptoms and complications of celiac disease, and additional treatment is needed. These individuals should schedule an appointment with their health care providers for an evaluation and to determine any additional steps they can take to recover their health.

If you accidentally eat a product that contains gluten, you may experience abdominal pain and diarrhea. Some people with celiac disease experience no signs or symptoms after eating gluten, but this doesn't mean the gluten isn't damaging the small intestine. Even consuming trace amounts of gluten can be damaging to someone with celiac disease, whether or not there are apparent symptoms afterward. Over time, not following a gluten-free diet can lead to serious complications, including cancer of the small intestine.

Replenish Nutrients

The nutrients that are absorbed by the jejunum (the area of the small intestine commonly affected by celiac disease) are amino acids, fatty acids, calcium, copper, iodine, iron, magnesium, phosphorus, potassium, zinc, and several vitamins (C, D, E, K, and most of the B vitamins). Consequently, there are many nutrients to consider replenishing when people with celiac disease are trying to restore their health. Nutritional healing is best accomplished by combining a diet rich in a wide variety of nutritious whole foods with a gluten-free dietary supplement. Since such a wide range of nutrients are involved, the regular use of a gluten-free multivitamin and mineral supplement is strongly recommended.

Because celiac disease involves inflammatory reactions, and because the absorption of fatty acids may be further reduced during flare-ups, it is important to pay special attention to your intake of omega-3 fatty acids. Ground flaxseeds and flaxseed oil are excellent, concentrated vegan sources of omega-3 fatty acids. If you use ground flaxseeds, you'll obtain not only the beneficial oil but also amino acids, fiber, and lignans, which will help soothe the damaged intestinal lining.

Other beneficial seeds and nuts to incorporate in your diet include almonds, Brazil nuts, chia seeds, hazelnuts, hemp seeds, pecans, pine nuts, pumpkin seeds, sesame seeds, sunflower seeds, and walnuts. Although seeds and nuts vary in their nutritional profiles and fat content, they all pack a lot of wholesome, healing nutrition into a tiny package.

Heal Damaged Intestines

When the digestive tract is healthy, it is able to filter out and eliminate damaging chemicals, harmful bacteria, toxins, and other waste products. Additionally, a healthy digestive tract takes in the things the body requires, including nutrients from food and water, and absorbs and helps deliver them to the cells where they are needed.

The digestive system normally has what is known as "good" bacteria and "bad" bacteria. Maintaining the correct balance between the good and the bad bacteria is necessary for optimal health. Poor food choices, emotional stress, lack of sleep, diseases (including celiac disease), antibiotic overuse, medications, and environmental influences can all shift the balance in favor of the bad bacteria.

The objective is not to destroy all of the bad bacteria; our bodies actually have a need for both kinds, good and bad. Problems arise, however, when the balance is shifted in the wrong direction and we end up with more of the bad bacteria than the good. An imbalance in the gut flora that results in an overgrowth of bad bacteria has been associated with diarrhea, fatigue, muscle pain, and urinary tract infections.

Because celiac disease imbalances the normal gut flora, restoring the intestines to good health is of prime importance. One of the most often recommended ways to do that is through the use of probiotics and prebiotics. Probiotics are gut-friendly microorganisms that help heal damaged intestines and restore the balance of the gut flora. Another critical way probiotics can help improve health is by strengthening the immune system. The immune system protects us from germs and diseases. When it isn't functioning properly, we are susceptible to allergic reactions, autoimmune disorders (such as Crohn's disease, rheumatoid arthritis, and ulcerative colitis), and infections (such as *Helicobacter pylori*, infectious diarrhea, skin infections, and vaginal infections).

Prebiotics are nondigestible carbohydrates that act as food for the probiotics. When probiotics and prebiotics work together, they form a synbiotic, or synergistic, relationship. Fermented foods, such as vegan yogurt, cultured vegetables (sauerkraut, kimchi, and pickles), fermented soy products (gluten-free tempeh and gluten-free miso), and fermented beverages (kombucha and KeVita brand sparkling probiotic drinks) contain active "friendly" bacteria. These foods are considered synbiotic because they contain both good bacteria and the fuel those bacteria need to thrive. Prebiotics are found in many whole foods, such as artichokes, asparagus, bananas, brown rice, garlic, leeks, legumes (beans, lentils, and peas), onions, and root vegetables. In addition, probiotics and prebiotics are added to some processed foods and are available as dietary supplements.

The Gluten-Free Diet

Since gluten is found only in grains, it's important to distinguish acceptable grains from unacceptable grains. In addition, avoiding wheat can be especially challenging because not only are wheat products and derivatives ubiquitous, but they also go by numerous names. The following list shows grains and related foods that contain gluten; these and any foods that contain them must be strictly avoided on a gluten-free diet.

Gluten-Containing Grains and Related Foods

- Barley
- Barley flour
- Bulgur
- Couscous
- Durum flour
- Einkorn
- Emmer
- Farina
- Farro
- Gluten
- Gluten flour
- Graham flour
- Groats
- High gluten flour
- Kamut *(khorasan wheat)*
- Modified food starch
- Oat bran *(unless certified GF)*
- Oat flour *(unless certified GF)*

- Oats *(unless certified GF)*
- Orzo
- Rye
- Rye flour
- Seitan
- Semolina
- Spelt
- Spelt flour
- Starch
- Triticale
- Vital wheat gluten
- Wheat
- Wheat bran
- Wheat flour
- Wheat germ
- Wheat gluten
- Wheat meat
- Wheat starch

Other Foods to Avoid

All the foods in the list of gluten-containing grains above are off limits with a gluten-free diet. If you're gluten sensitive, take care to avoid all wheat-containing items and all gluten-containing grains and products made from them or that contain them. With a straightforward wheat allergy, a number of the items in the gluten-containing list may be appropriate if they are explicitly from a non-wheat source. However, people with celiac disease need to be extra vigilant because the source of a questionable ingredient may be wheat or other gluten-containing grains. For example, a wheat-sensitive person may be able to tolerate malt made from barley, but a gluten-sensitive person cannot because barley is a prohibited grain that contains gluten. Unfortunately, the statement "wheat-free" on a food label does not necessarily mean "gluten-free." Below is a list of many common food items that sometimes or always contain gluten but not necessarily wheat. In general, avoid these foods unless they're specifically labeled as gluten-free and it's clear that they're made with corn, rice, other gluten-free grains, or soy:

- Ales
- Baked beans, canned
- Barley malt
- Beers
- Bread crumbs
- Breaded foods
- Breads
- Brewer's yeast
- Cakes
- Candies
- Cereals
- Coffee alternatives
- Communion wafers
- Cookies
- Cracker meal
- Crackers
- Croutons
- Dried dates dusted with flour
- Energy bars
- Farina
- Faux meats
- Flavored coffees
- Flavored teas
- French fries
- Fried vegetables
- Frozen entrées
- Granola bars
- Gravies
- Gravy mixes
- Hot chocolate mix
- Hydrolyzed wheat protein
- Instant hot drinks
- Ketchup
- Lagers
- Malt
- Malt extract
- Malt flavoring
- Malt syrup
- Malt vinegar
- Malted liquor
- Marinades
- Matzo
- Nondairy creamers
- Nondairy milks with malt
- Noodles
- Pastas
- Pickles
- Pies
- Potato chips
- Ready-to-eat entrées
- Roasted nuts
- Root beer
- Salad dressings
- Sauces
- Seasoned rice mixes
- Seasoned snacks foods
- Seitan
- Soup bases
- Soups
- Soy sauce
- Soymilk
- Syrups
- Tabbouleh

- Tempura vegetables
- Teriyaki sauce
- Tortilla chips
- Trail mix
- Vegan imitation seafood
- Vegetable bouillon cubes
- Vegetable protein
- Vegetables in sauce
- Veggie bacon
- Veggie burgers
- Veggie dogs
- Veggie meats
- Veggie sausage
- Vodka
- Wine coolers

Miscellaneous Sources of Gluten

In addition to foods, you should be alert for other products that you eat or that could come in contact with your mouth that may contain gluten. These include the following:

- Bakeries (airborne gluten)
- Bulk bins
- Cosmetics
- Lip balms
- Lip gloss
- Lipsticks
- Medications
- Mineral supplements
- Non-self-adhesive envelopes
- Non-self-adhesive stamps
- Play-Doh
- Shampoos
- Supplements (check label)
- Vitamins (check label)

Gluten-Free Grains and Related Foods

The following list includes grains that are naturally gluten-free and are therefore acceptable on a gluten-free diet. Nonetheless, be aware that although these grains and foods are gluten-free by nature, they could potentially contain gluten due to cross-contamination with gluten-containing grains (see "Watch Out for Cross-Contamination," page 13). For people with gluten sensitivity who can tolerate minute amounts of gluten, this isn't of particular concern; for people with celiac disease, however, it's crucial. Also note that despite its name, buckwheat, pure buckwheat flour, and 100 percent buckwheat soba noodles are naturally gluten-free. Still, many products labeled "buckwheat flour" might contain buckwheat as well as wheat or other gluten-containing flours. Always read labels carefully.

- Almond flour
- Amaranth
- Amaranth flour
- Arrowroot starch
- Bean flours
- Buckwheat flour
- Buckwheat groats (kasha)
- Chia seeds
- Chickpea flour
- Coconut flour
- Corn
- Corn flour
- Cornmeal
- Cornstarch
- Distilled alcoholic beverages
- Distilled vinegars
- Flaxseeds
- Gluten-free pasta
- Hominy (corn)
- Job's tears
- Millet
- Millet flour
- Pea flour
- Polenta (corn grits)
- Potato flour
- Potato starch
- Quinoa
- Quinoa flakes
- Quinoa flour
- Rice (all varieties)
- Rice flour
- Rice pasta
- Sorghum (milo)
- Sorghum flour
- Soy flour
- Tapioca flour
- Tapioca starch
- Taro
- Teff
- Wild rice

Food Labeling

In January 2006, the Food Allergen Labeling and Consumer Protection Act (FALCPA) took effect. This act requires specific labels for food products that contain major food allergens, such as milk, eggs, fish, crustacean shellfish, peanuts, tree nuts, wheat, and soy. Products covered by FALCPA include conventional foods, dietary supplements, infant formula, and medical foods. The allergen must be noted in plain language, either in the ingredient list or via the word "Contains" followed by the name of the major food allergen. For example, a label might state, "Contains eggs, wheat." Alternatively, it might be in the ingredient list in parentheses, such as "lecithin (soy)" or "enriched flour (wheat flour, malted barley)." Such ingredients must be listed if they are present in any amount, even in food colorings, flavors, or spice blends. Also, manufacturers must list the specific nut (for example, almond, cashew, or walnut) or seafood (for example, tuna, salmon, shrimp, or lobster) that is used.

Although FALCPA has made reading labels easier and more useful, it doesn't cover gluten, only wheat. Therefore, it's critical to read all labels on all packages carefully every time. Ingredients and manufacturing processes can change without warning, so reading labels each time you shop will help ensure that you're buying products that are safe for you.

The use of advisory labeling, including precautionary statements such as "may contain," "processed in a facility that also processes," or "made on equipment with," is voluntary and optional for manufacturers. There currently are no laws governing or requiring these statements, so they may or may not indicate whether a product contains a specific allergen. According to the Food and Drug Administration's guidance to the food industry on this issue, advisory labels "should not be used as a substitute for adhering to current good manufacturing practices and must be truthful and not misleading." If you are unsure whether a product could be contaminated with gluten, you should call the manufacturer to ask about the ingredients used and the company's processing practices prior to your buying the product.

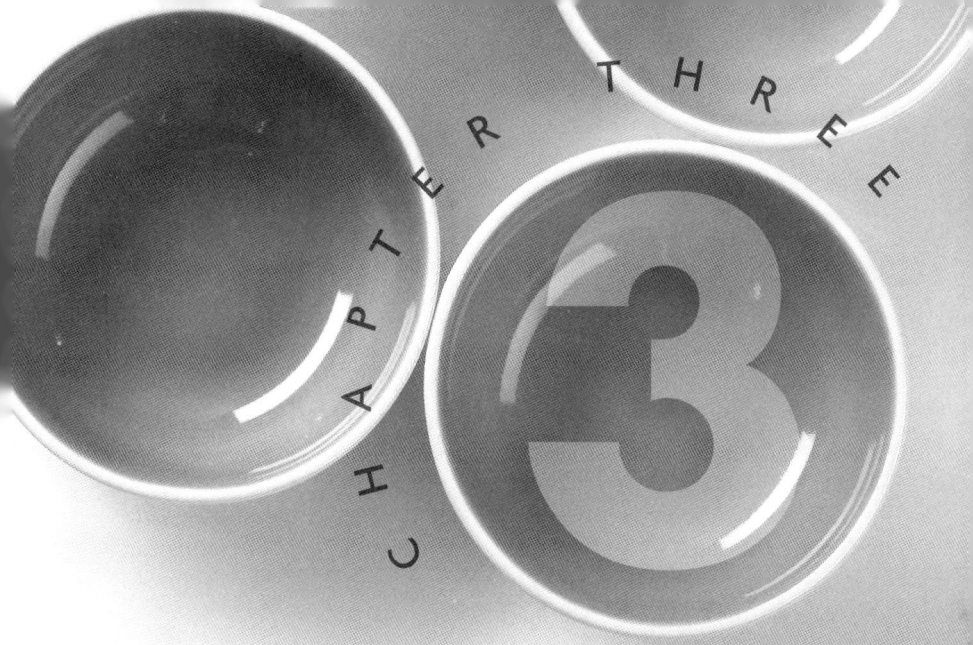

Watch Out for Cross-Contamination

C ross-contamination occurs when foods that would normally be gluten-free come into contact with foods that contain gluten. For example, this can happen during the manufacturing process if the same equipment is used to make other products that contain wheat or gluten.

Some food labels include a "may contain" statement if cross-contamination is likely. Nevertheless, bear in mind that this type of labeling is voluntary and not all manufacturers use it for potentially cross-contaminated products. Food products may also be labeled as "gluten-free." For foods that carry this label, the Food and Drug Administration requires that they contain less than twenty parts per million (20 ppm) of gluten. Be aware that products labeled "wheat-free" may still contain gluten. Of course, it's essential that you check the actual ingredient list. If you're not sure whether a food contains gluten, don't buy it, or check with the manufacturer first to inquire about what it contains. The best mantra to follow is "when in doubt, go without."

It's extremely important to also be careful when eating out at restaurants. Ask the waitstaff if the restaurant has truly gluten-free vegan options and whether the chef and kitchen crew take measures when preparing the food so that cross-contamination is avoided. (See "Dining Out Safely," page 16.)

Cross-contamination can also occur at home. If foods are prepared on common surfaces or with utensils that weren't thoroughly cleaned after being used to prepare gluten-containing foods, cross-contamination is inevitable. Sharing a toaster for gluten-free bread and regular bread, for example, or sharing common kitchen items, such as baking sheets, colanders, dish towels, and utensils, demonstrates how gluten contamination can easily occur. Evaluate your circumstances and determine the steps you need to take to prevent cross-contamination at home, school, or work. Following are some practical strategies to help you prevent cross-contamination:

Buying Food

- Buy prepackaged gluten-free grains and other products.

  Look for grains and other products that are certified gluten-free and noted as such on the label to ensure cross-contamination didn't take place during processing.

- Buy prepackaged gluten-free flours.

  Purchase only flours that are labeled as being gluten-free, and buy only those that are manufactured by reputable companies, as they are more likely to test for gluten. Look for well-sealed plastic, aseptic, or metal packaging, since products in unlined paper can become contaminated if they're stored near wheat or shipped in the same trucks that transport wheat.

- Avoid purchasing imported foods.

  Imported foods are risky because other countries may not abide by the same gluten-free standards as the United States.

- Steer clear of the bulk bins.

  Don't buy unpackaged foods stored in the supermarket bulk bins or bulk bins at the natural food store. The bins may have previously held gluten-containing foods and may not have been cleaned adequately. In addition, the scoops used to put the foods in bags or containers may have also been used with nearby gluten-containing foods.

Storing Food

■ **Store foods separately.**

Keep gluten-free products on the top shelf of the pantry or refrigerator so other foods don't accidentally drip or drop down and cross-contaminate them.

■ **Prevent double dipping.**

Buy squeezable condiment containers for ketchup, mustard, and mayonnaise to prevent double dipping.

■ **Color-code food.**

Use different-colored stickers to distinguish between gluten-containing and gluten-free products in the pantry and refrigerator.

Preparing Food

■ **Avoid wooden utensils.**

Don't use wooden spoons or cutting boards that also are used to prepare gluten-containing foods. Wood can harbor residual gluten. Metal, plastic, and silicone are better choices.

■ **Use different-colored equipment.**

Purchase equipment in various colors to distinguish what it's used for. For example, purchase a colander in a different color for gluten-free foods so it doesn't get mixed up with the colander used for gluten-containing foods.

■ **Buy separate appliances.**

Buy separate blenders, stick blenders, food processors, toasters, waffle makers, and bread-making machines if the ones you currently have don't have parts that can be disassembled and put in the dishwasher.

■ **Segregate areas of the grill.**

Have clearly defined areas of the barbecue grill for gluten-free foods when sharing grilling surfaces. Cover areas of the grill that were used for gluten-containing foods (or that you suspect might have been) before grilling gluten-free ones.

■ **Provide safe party foods.**

When planning a dinner party or buffet, prepare foods that are completely free of gluten to prevent accidental cross-contamination among family members and guests. Don't serve food that others have brought unless it's prepackaged and you're certain it's safe. Avoid attending potluck gatherings and buffets in restaurants or other people's homes, where you can't control how the food is prepared or served, because cross-contamination (even with the gluten-free food you've provided) is likely to occur.

Dining Out Safely

When you initially go gluten-free—whether as part of a trial elimination diet to determine gluten sensitivity or after a diagnosis of celiac disease—it's a good idea to avoid eating out for a few months to be sure you don't accidentally ingest gluten and derail your progress. This will also give you time to become comfortable with the diet and with explaining your needs to restaurant staff when you do start eating out again. Always do advance research before dining out so you can rest assured that your food will be safe for you and you can enjoy your meal without worry.

Talk to the owners of your favorite restaurants as well as the chefs and waitstaff about your dietary restrictions so they understand the seriousness of this issue. Explain which foods you can and can't eat, and make sure the kitchen team knows how to avoid cross-contamination. If you're not satisfied with the responses you receive, take your business elsewhere.

When selecting a restaurant, pay attention to the size and breadth of the menu. If it's huge and contains countless selections, it's likely that processed ingredients are used and the dishes are assembled in advance rather than made to order. Look for restaurants that have limited menus with a focus on fresh ingredients.

Soups and sauces are typically thickened with wheat flour, so always inquire about the thickeners that are used in them. Ask about coatings and breading on vegan proteins (such as tempeh and tofu) and vegetables. If you're considering anything fried, ask whether the fryer is used for foods coated with flour, bread crumbs, or other wheat products. Don't avoid asking about ingredients in marinades, rubs, salad dressings, seasonings, spices, and marinades. Remember that surprising ingredients, such as soy sauce and chili powder, can contain wheat. Many Asian restaurants have wheat-free tamari instead of soy sauce, so don't be shy about asking for it. Heat doesn't destroy gluten, so if you order something grilled, ask that the grill be thoroughly cleaned before your food is cooked on it. Better yet, ask if the food can be baked instead of grilled or fried.

If you're not comfortable speaking to restaurant staff openly, or if you're traveling and there's a language barrier, order and carry dining cards (such as those from celiactravel.com or glutenfreepassport.com) that will communicate your dietary needs and make it clear that this is a serious condition, not a preference.

Online and local in-person support groups can help you find good, safe eating spots in your area. They can also be great for people learning to cope with celiac disease and for finding (and becoming) an advocate. Check out celiac.com for a list of support groups throughout the world.

The Oat Controversy

A large body of scientific evidence has been accumulated over the last few decades showing that oats are well tolerated by the vast majority of people with celiac disease. Botanically, oats are not related to gluten-containing grains, such as wheat, barley, and rye, and they don't contain gluten. Instead, they contain proteins called avenins, which are nontoxic and usually not problematic for individuals with celiac disease or gluten sensitivity.

Oats are a rotation crop with wheat, barley, and rye, and as most farmers eventually discover, "volunteer" plants will occasionally shoot up among the alternating crop if they had been planted in the field the previous year. Consequently, oats can become contaminated with wheat, barley, or rye directly in the field as well as by the equipment used to harvest and process these grains. In this all-too-common scenario, cross-contamination isn't preventable, and therefore these "regular" oats are not safe to eat by anyone with celiac disease. Keep in mind that individuals with gluten sensitivity (not celiac disease) may be able to tolerate minute amounts of gluten. If you fall into that category, "regular" oats should be fine for you; however, if you have celiac disease or find that even microscopic amounts of gluten cause symptoms, look for oats that are certified gluten-free instead.

Certified gluten-free oats are grown in a fashion similar to organic crops. For starters, a field must lay fallow for least four years, which eliminates the possibility of volunteer plants. All harvesting and processing equipment must be used solely for the production of oats. And, finally, the oats must be certified as being gluten-free. This process requires that national gluten-intolerance certifying organizations inspect and test the oats and the facility in which they are processed to ensure the above steps are followed and that the oats meet the US standard for gluten-free, which is less than twenty parts per million (20 ppm).

Oats can be an important part of a gluten-free diet provided they are selected from sources that guarantee a lack of contamination by wheat, barley, or rye. If oats are well tolerated, they can be a valuable and nutrient-rich addition to a diet that's generally limited in other grains. If you're not certain whether you can tolerate oats, you may want to introduce certified gluten-free oats into your diet in small amounts and keep a detailed food diary to track your responses.

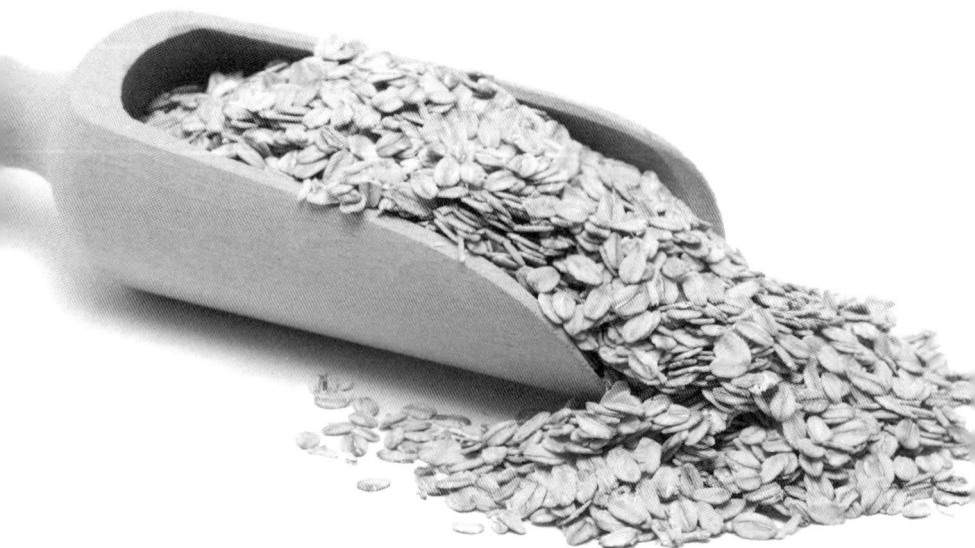

Gluten-Free
Cooking Basics

Getting Started

G luten-free cooking can be challenging at first, mainly because it's something new and different that must be dealt with several times a day. However, it's not essential to use special gluten-free products unless you really want to. You'll actually have the most success if you keep your cooking and your meals uncomplicated and stick with recipes and ingredients that are basic and familiar.

Begin by focusing on simple, whole, gluten-free foods with no additives. Basing meals on straightforward items such as fresh fruits, vegetables, beans, nuts, seeds, and plain tofu is an excellent place to start. Vegetables and fruits are naturally gluten-free and packed with great nutrition. Starchier foods, such as potatoes, sweet potatoes, and winter squashes, make ideal foundations for hearty meals. Gluten-free grain choices include rice and risotto, corn and polenta, buckwheat, millet, and quinoa. White and yellow corn tortillas are terrific for making Mexican dishes such as enchiladas, fajitas, and tacos. Brown rice tortillas are handy for making burritos, roll-ups, and wraps, and they can even be used as a superquick base for a thin-crust, gluten-free pizza. There are some outstanding gluten-free pastas on the market made from various grains, such as amaranth, brown rice, corn, and quinoa, and traditional Asian rice noodles are also gluten-free. Rice paper wrappers (used to make fresh spring rolls) are usually gluten-free; wonton wrappers are not, as they are made from wheat. Starches and thickeners for gluten-free cooking include arrowroot, cornstarch, potato starch, tapioca, and tapioca starch. Chickpea flour is useful for thickening gravies and sauces.

When done right, gluten-free cooking doesn't have to be overly restrictive or isolating, and it can definitely be fun, enjoyable, and delicious. Below is a list of useful substitutes for common foods that contain gluten. Using these and similar alternatives will streamline your cooking and enable you to follow many conventional recipes while

Common gluten-containing foods and suitable alternatives

GLUTEN-CONTAINING ITEMS	ALTERNATIVES
Barley	Brown rice
Bulgur	Quinoa
Couscous, pearl	Sorghum
Couscous, regular	Quinoa or millet
Flour tortillas	Brown rice tortillas or gluten-free corn tortillas
Rolled oats, standard	Certified gluten-free rolled oats, rice flakes, or quinoa flakes
Seitan ("wheat meat")	Tempeh,* baked tofu, or legumes (beans, lentils, or peas)
Semolina or durum wheat pasta	Rice, corn, or quinoa pasta
Soy sauce	Wheat-free soy sauce, wheat-free tamari, Bragg Liquid Aminos, or gluten-free miso
Tofu, seasoned	Tofu, plain
Udon noodles	Rice linguine or 100 percent buckwheat soba noodles
Worcestershire sauce	The Wizard's Organic GF/CF Worcestershire Sauce, Bragg Liquid Aminos, or gluten-free miso thinned with a little water

* Tempeh may be made with gluten-containing ingredients, such as soy sauce or wheat grain. Choose an unflavored, unseasoned, 100 percent soy tempeh, and carefully check the label.

keeping them gluten-free. Remember to always check labels for possible gluten-containing ingredients and additives.

Gluten-Free Grains

Going gluten-free doesn't mean you have to go grain-free. Even if you're able to tolerate gluten, it's worth exploring the variety of nutritious and great-tasting gluten-free grains available, including amaranth, buckwheat, corn, millet, quinoa, rice, sorghum, teff, and wild rice, among others. These grains have a long and honorable history. Corn was grown in Mexico seven thousand years ago. Millet was among the first grains to be cultivated, with records dating back to 5500 BC in China and even earlier in Africa. Amaranth was harvested for thousands of years by Mayan and Incan civilizations. Quinoa, grown for five thousand years in the South American Andes Mountains, was called "the mother grain" by the Incas because it was believed to impart long life.

Although they're seldom regarded as protein providers, grains supply half the world's protein. Most whole grains have an ideal balance of protein, fat, and carbohydrates, as well as a full complement of trace minerals, such as chromium, iron, magnesium, selenium, and zinc, along with B vitamins. B vitamins work in concert to release the food energy that's stored in whole grains. In contrast, refined grains have been stripped of the majority of their nutrients. Although refined grains are often fortified with some of the nutrients that are lost in processing (notably several B vitamins and iron), the vast majority of the nutrients (such as calcium, fiber, magnesium, selenium, vitamin C, and zinc) are gone forever.

From a nutritional perspective, whole grains are particularly beneficial for people with celiac disease because the fiber positively affects intestinal flora and provides support for friendly intestinal bacteria. Whole grains modulate the glycemic response, meaning that they deliver energy in a gentle and gradual manner. They are also rich in antioxidants and protective against cardiovascular disease and cancers of the gastrointestinal tract. Another welcome advantage of gluten-free grains is that most of them, other than brown rice and wild rice, cook fairly quickly.

Meet the Gluten-Free Whole-Grain All-Stars

The following list includes nutrient-rich, gluten-free grains that would be valuable for everyone (gluten-free or not) to include in their culinary repertoire:

AMARANTH. Cooked like a grain, amaranth is actually the seed of a plant that is native to Central and South America. Amaranth is a source of complete protein; it contains all the essential amino acids, including lysine, which is lacking in most grains. High in fiber and a good source of magnesium and iron, amaranth is a spectacular addition to any diet. Amaranth has an earthy, nutty flavor, and uncooked amaranth can be cooked and used in gluten-free breads and baked goods to boost nutrition and impart a crunchy texture. It can also be cooked into a porridge, used to make amaranth polenta, or added to soups.

BUCKWHEAT. A nutritional powerhouse, buckwheat is a mainstay of traditional Eastern European cuisine and the star of many classic dishes from that region of the world. Buckwheat groats are the hulled, triangular seeds of the buckwheat plant, a relative of rhubarb and sorrel. These soft white seeds have a mild flavor, but when they're toasted or roasted, the flavor becomes rich and intense. Roasted buckwheat groats are known as kasha. Buckwheat groats can be cooked like rice and used in pilafs, casseroles, salads, and side dishes. If you're so inclined, you can ground the groats in your own mill to make fresh buckwheat flour. Buckwheat provides complete protein, including all the essential amino acids, and is a good source of calcium, copper, magnesium, niacin, and riboflavin.

CORN. Although most people think of corn as a vegetable, served on the cob or popped, there are other forms of corn that are particularly valuable to people on a gluten-free diet. When corn is dried, it can be ground into a coarse or fine meal or flour. It can also be made into pasta, on its own or combined with other gluten-free grains. Coarse cornmeal (grits) is used to make traditional cornbread, a staple in the South, and polenta, an Italian specialty. Although corn is relatively low in protein, it contains fiber, vitamin B_6 (pyridoxine), and selenium.

MILLET. An ancient grain from the Far East, millet was first farmed nearly ten thousand years ago. It was revered as one of five sacred crops in ancient China and is mentioned in the Old Testament, the writings of Herodotus, and the journals of Marco Polo. Millet has a mild, sweet flavor and a quick cooking time, making it a tasty, convenient, whole-grain addition to any meal of the day. Unlike most other grains, versatile millet is alkaline, which makes it easy to digest and helps balance the body's natural tendency toward acidity. Millet is an excellent source of dietary fiber and is rich in the B vitamins folate, riboflavin, and thiamine. Whole-grain millet makes a delicious alternative to rice in salads and stir-fries. To replace mashed potatoes, cook millet with a little extra water and serve it with a drizzle of olive oil and a dash of salt and pepper. Millet can also be cooked into a sweet breakfast porridge, and uncooked millet can be added to gluten-free bread dough for a crunchy texture.

QUINOA. A staple of the ancient Incas, quinoa (pronounced KEEN-wah) was revered because it was one of the few crops that could survive in such high altitudes and withstand frost, intense sun, and the often dry conditions that characterized the Andean climate. It was also recognized for its superior nutritional qualities. Technically quinoa isn't a grain but the seed of a plant in the same family as lamb's quarters. In cooking, however, it's used like a whole grain. Quinoa is an excellent source of complete protein, providing all the essential amino acids. It is also a good source of dietary fiber. Quinoa's light, earthy flavor and delightful texture make it ideal for pilafs, soups, and salads. Unlike brown rice and gluten-containing whole grains, quinoa takes relatively little time to cook and can be used as a substitute for other whole grains in almost any recipe. It's also a nutritious alternative to couscous and white rice in most dishes. Quinoa usually needs to be rinsed before using to remove a naturally occurring resin called saponin that coats its grains. However, some brands of quinoa are prerinsed and will state that on the package, making the rinsing step unnecessary. Both whole quinoa and quinoa flakes can be cooked into a tasty hot breakfast cereal (see pages 65 and 68). Quinoa pasta is readily available in a variety of shapes and sizes.

RICE. Rice has fed more people over a longer period of time than any other crop known to humankind. It tends to be a mainstay of gluten-free, nonallergenic diets and is available in many varieties. Long-grain rice cooks up to be dry and fluffy, with distinct individual grains; short-grain rice is soft and sticky; and medium-grain rice has attributes of both the long and short varieties. Long- and medium-grain rices are generally used for main courses, while short-grain rice is used for risottos, desserts, and Japanese foods, such as nori rolls, that require sticky rice. Basmati rice is a unique, aromatic strain that is grown in the foothills of the Himalayas. Jasmine rice is an aromatic long-grain rice that's been grown in the mountain highlands of Thailand for centuries; it was first cultivated for the royalty of the kingdom of Siam. And there are a variety of specialty rices from around the world that you can explore, such as arborio rice from Italy, red rice from Camargue in southern France, red rice from Bhutan, black forbidden rice (also known as purple rice) from China, pink rice from Madagascar, and many others that are fragrant or have distinctive colors. Brown rice and white rice are also available in a wide range of pastas.

SORGHUM. Sorghum originated in Africa thousands of years ago and made its way through the Middle East and Asia via ancient trade routes, traveling to the Arabian Peninsula, India, and China along the Silk Road. Today sorghum remains a staple food in India and Africa, yet it's still relatively unknown in most other parts of the world. This naturally gluten-free grain is an excellent source of dietary fiber and has a hearty, chewy texture similar to wheat berries, making it an ideal addition to pilafs and cold salads. Replace noodles or white rice in soups with sorghum for a more nutritious alternative. Sorghum can also be popped like popcorn in a microwave or on the stove top.

TEFF. A tiny grain that has been a staple of traditional Ethiopian cooking for thousands of years, whole-grain teff is a nutritional powerhouse. An ancient East African cereal grass, teff is the smallest grain in the world; it takes about one hundred grains of teff to equal the size of a single wheat berry! The germ and bran, where the nutrients are concentrated, account for a larger volume of the seed compared to more common grains. Teff has a mild, nutty flavor and is packed with calcium, protein, and fiber. It makes a terrific addition to hot cereals, stews, pilafs, or gluten-free baked goods. Whole-grain teff can be cooked into a unique porridge, similar in texture and consistency to wheat farina. Teff can also be made into a teff-based polenta, added to veggie burgers and casseroles, or mixed into batters for gluten-free cakes, cookies, and breads. Teff flour is the main ingredient in the popular fermented Ethiopian bread *injera*. Be aware, however, that commercial *injera* and *injera* sold at Ethiopian restaurants typically contains wheat as well as teff, so be sure to ask in advance and always read labels carefully before ordering or purchasing.

WILD RICE. Native to the United States and parts of Canada, wild rice isn't really a rice at all but a long-grain marsh grass. It has almost twice the protein content of rice and a higher proportion of protein than many other whole grains. Wild rice is unusually rich in the mineral zinc, is high in the B vitamins niacin and folate, and is a good source of calcium and iron. It has a delicious, nutty flavor when cooked alone or mixed with brown rice. Wild rice will enhance the flavor of any meal, from the simple to the gourmet.

Tips for Preparing Gluten-Free Whole Grains

You can easily add more gluten-free grains to your meals simply by choosing gluten-free vegan breads, breakfast cereals, and pastas. However, there's nothing quite as pleasurable and satisfying as eating whole, natural grains that haven't been refined in any way. Whole grains are usually chewier than refined grains and have a nuttier, fuller flavor. To enjoy delicious whole grains at home in a main dish or side dish, use the guidelines that follow for cooking them from scratch.

Cooking most gluten-free whole grains is very similar to cooking rice. Simply put the dry grain in a saucepan with water or vegetable broth, bring to a boil, decrease the heat to low, cover, and simmer until the liquid is absorbed. To make a pilaf instead of plain grain, brown small amounts of chopped onion, mushrooms, and/or garlic in a little oil in a saucepan. Add the grain and toast it briefly, coating the grains with the flavored oil. Then add the proper amount of water or broth (see the table on page 26) and cook until the liquid is absorbed and the grain is tender.

Grains can vary in cooking time depending on the age of the grain, the variety of grain, and the pan you're using to cook it in, so adjust the amount of liquid used and the cooking time as needed. When you decide the grain is tender and tasty, it's done. If the grain is not as soft as you'd like when the cooking time has ended, simply add more water and continue cooking. Or, if the grain is tender before all the liquid is absorbed, simply drain the excess liquid.

To cook grain even more quickly (although most gluten-free whole grains take very little time), let it sit in the allotted amount of water for a few hours before cooking. When you're ready to cook it, add a little extra water if necessary. You'll find that the cooking time will be decreased quite a bit. Another time-saving trick is to cook whole grains in big batches. Cooked grains will keep for three to four days in the refrigerator and take mere minutes to warm up with a little added water or vegetable broth. Use leftover cooked grain as the base for cold salads; just toss the grain with chopped vegetables and gluten-free vegan salad dressing. Leftover cooked grain also makes a pleasing addition to leftover soup; and best of all, you can warm up the grain and soup together right in the same pot.

Sometimes gluten-free whole grain will stick to the bottom of the saucepan during cooking. If that happens, simply turn off the heat or remove the pan from the heat, add a very small amount of water, broth, or other liquid, cover the pan with a lid, and let the grain sit for a few minutes. The stuck grain will steam and loosen, making serving and cleanup a whole lot easier.

Cooking times for common gluten-free whole grains

GRAIN (1 CUP)	WATER OR VEGETABLE BROTH	COOKING TIME	YIELD
Amaranth	2 cups	20 to 25 minutes	3½ cups
Buckwheat groats	2 cups	20 minutes	4 cups
Cornmeal, coarse (polenta; yellow corn grits)	4 cups	15 to 20 minutes	2½ cups
Millet, hulled*	2½ cups	25 to 35 minutes	4 cups
Oats, steel cut	4 cups	25 to 35 minutes	4 cups
Quinoa	1½ cups	25 minutes	3 cups
Rice, brown	2½ cups	35 to 50 minutes (depending on variety)	3 to 4 cups
Sorghum	3 cups	55 to 65 minutes	3 cups
Wild rice**	3 cups	50 to 60 minutes	3½ cups

* Millet will taste best if it is toasted before cooking. Put it in the saucepan and heat over medium-high heat, stirring frequently, until it turns a rich golden brown and the grains are fragrant, 4 to 5 minutes. Be careful not to let the grains burn. Because the saucepan will be hot, the water will sputter when you pour it in, so stand back.

** Wild rice is cooked when the kernels puff open and are butterflied. If they are done cooking before all the water is absorbed, drain the excess liquid and let the rice rest, covered, for 5 to 10 minutes.

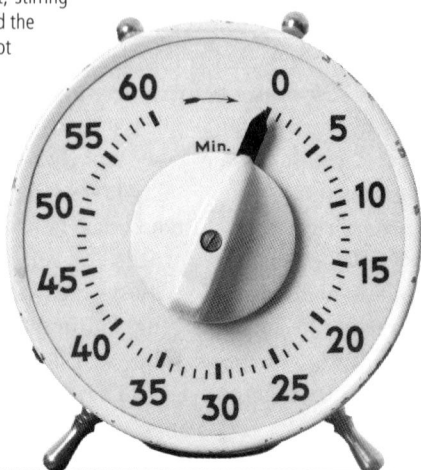

CHAPTER FIVE

Gluten-Free Baking Basics

It's true that baking is as much a science as an art, and there's no question that baking without gluten can be a challenge. Wheat gluten gives elasticity to baked goods in a way that no other single grain can replicate. Without gluten, baked goods can be gummy, heavy bricks. The most satisfying, tender, and delicious gluten-free recipes employ a mixture of grains along with some texturizing ingredients, such as tapioca, to help mimic the elastic qualities of wheat flour and provide the chewy mouthfeel of products that are made with it. To ensure a positive gluten-free baking experience, adhere to the tips that follow and you'll be turning out perfect gluten-free baked goods in no time.

Tips for Perfect Gluten-Free Baked Goods

One of the many food-related questions that people newly diagnosed with celiac disease and gluten sensitivity commonly ask is whether they'll ever be able to have bread, cake, or other baked goods again. Fortunately, the answer is a resounding yes. Just be sure to follow the recipe directions carefully and always use the exact ingredients called for. With gluten-free baking mixes now readily available, even in mainstream supermarkets, and with abundant vegan alternatives for eggs, it's become surprisingly easy to have your gluten-free cake and eat it too. Here are some tips for a positive and successful gluten-free baking experience:

Ingredients

- **Don't sample raw batter.**
  Gluten-free batters typically contain uncooked bean flours and other ingredients that can cause severe gastrointestinal upset. Although the finished baked goods are delicious, the batters generally do not taste very good before they are baked.

- **Use fresh baking powder.**
  Be sure the baking powder you have is fresh (check the expiration date on the container), as it will lose its leavening power over time. To test if your baking powder is still active, stir 1 teaspoon of it into ⅓ cup of hot water. If it bubbles vigorously, it is fine. Note that although some baking powders produced in the United Kingdom may contain wheat starch, nowadays virtually all baking powders produced in the United States use cornstarch (or sometimes potato starch), which is gluten-free. However, as with all products, read the label carefully before purchasing to be on the safe side.

- **Adjust liquid as needed.**
  Gluten-free flours and mixes will vary in their moisture content from batch to batch because of uncontrollable variables with cultivation, harvesting, and storage of the primary flour ingredients. As a result, at times you may need to add slightly more or less liquid than is called for in a recipe.

- **Use xanthan gum or guar gum.**
  Most gluten-free baked goods fare better if a small amount of xanthan gum or guar gum is added to the dry ingredients. The gum replicates some of the properties of gluten-containing grains by helping gluten-free baked goods hold together better. Generally, ¼ to ½ teaspoon of xanthan gum or guar gum is recommended for each cup of gluten-free all-purpose flour when it's being used

to replace wheat flour in conventional recipes. Note that guar gum can cause diarrhea in some people; if you're sensitive to it, use xanthan gum instead.

- **Learn to balance flavors.**

Recipes calling for a blend of flours tend to have a more balanced flavor and a more tender crumb than those that rely on only one type of flour. As you become more comfortable with gluten-free baking, experiment with various gluten-free flours to learn the flavors and textures that various types contribute and which ones you prefer.

- **Store ingredients properly.**

Many gluten-free flours, especially those made with legumes, nuts, and whole grains, are higher in fat than standard wheat flour and can spoil more readily. Check expiration dates and store higher-fat gluten-free flours in the freezer to prolong their freshness.

Preparation and Equipment

- **Use the correct baking pan.**

Always use the type and size of pan called for in each recipe. A too-small pan can cause a gluten-free cake to overflow while baking or to not cook properly in the center; a pan that's too big may cause the cake to burn. The only exception to this is bread; baking gluten-free breads in slightly smaller loaf pans encourages a higher rise and a tastier crust.

- **Use metal bakeware.**

For more even baking, use a metal baking pan or cookie sheet. Other materials, such as glass or ceramic, heat faster than metal and can cause gluten-free baked goods to become overcooked on the outside and undercooked in the interior.

- **Oil pans properly.**

When a recipe directs you to oil a pan, you'll get the best results with a gluten-free nonhydrogenated vegetable shortening or coconut oil. Organic or virgin coconut oil can be found in natural food stores or online.

- **Try parchment paper or nonstick baking mats.**

Parchment paper and reusable silicone baking mats (such as Silpat brand) are great for lining baking sheets and pans. They eliminate the need to oil bakeware and make cleanup a pleasure. Alternatively, use well-oiled or nonstick bakeware.

- **Sift gluten-free flours before using.**

  When mixing dry ingredients for cakes, cookies, quick breads, and other baked goods, you will achieve a lighter product if you sift the flours first. As old-fashioned as this might sound, adding a bit of air to gluten-free flours makes baked items more tender and gives them a better crumb.

- **Avoid tough dough.**

  With standard wheat dough, overbeating can make the finished product tough; that's because beating makes the gluten bonds stronger and more elastic. Contrarily, most gluten-free doughs benefit from being beaten for several minutes because this process will aerate and lighten them. Using a heavy-duty stand mixer rather than a handheld mixer will make the process easier.

- **Oil or moisten hands with water.**

  Gluten-free doughs and batters can get very sticky. Using oiled or wet hands will greatly help with keeping the mixture from sticking to them.

Baking, Cooling, and Storing

- **Set the oven temperature precisely.**

  If necessary, get an oven thermometer to check your oven's temperature if you think it might need to be calibrated. An inaccurate oven temperature can ruin any baked good.

- **Watch baking times closely.**

  Small changes, such as substituting ingredients or not measuring accurately, can cause even the most wonderful recipe to fail. Baking times will fluctuate if you vary the ingredients, aren't careful with your measurements, or use a different type or size of pan than what is called for in the recipe.

- **Preheat the oven.**

  Always preheat the oven to the temperature specified. Batters for quick breads (those that contain baking powder rather than yeast) will not keep well while waiting until the oven is ready. Work quickly with recipes that contain baking powder. These recipes must be baked immediately or the baking powder will lose much of its punch and the baked goods will be flat or have a poor rise.

- **Prevent mushiness.**

  Gluten-free baked goods can become mushy if they emit too much steam while baking, and because gluten-free dough is usually moister than conventional wheat-based dough, this can easily happen. Pizza stones can help remedy this and are essential for baking crisp breads, crackers, and pizza crusts. Another method is to remove breads from their loaf pans when they are firm enough to hold their shape (about two-thirds of the way through baking) and then finish baking them directly on the oven rack or on a preheated pizza stone.

- **Cool completely.**

  Cool quick breads completely before slicing or wrapping them to avoid a gummy texture.

- **Store baked goods properly.**

  Gluten-free muffins, cakes, and quick breads will keep for one to two days at room temperature. After that, store them loosely wrapped in the refrigerator. Most can also be frozen for up to three months (cakes should be frozen without frosting). Cookies, crackers, and biscuits can be stored at room temperature.

Key Ingredients for Gluten-Free Baking

Gluten-free baking has never been easier or tastier. Increased interest in alternative and minimally refined grains has revolutionized the major ingredients used in most gluten-free baked goods. Rice flour reigns supreme, but it generally has a gritty texture and lower nutritional profile compared to other flours. Today a broad selection of options abound, including gluten-free grain flours, nut flours, and legume flours, as well as superfine rice flour, which has been milled on a very fine setting to eliminate grittiness. Although rice flour remains the queen of gluten-free baking, when it's combined with other gluten-free flours and starches, the nutrition of baked goods is boosted and the texture is smoothed. Following is a list of some of the essential ingredients that modern gluten-free bakers use to create healthy, delicious recipes.

Gluten-free flours and essential baking ingredients

INGREDIENT	ATTRIBUTES
Almond flour	Sweet, nutty flavor; high in fat and protein; store in the refrigerator or freezer
Amaranth flour	High in protein; distinctive taste and texture; best used in combination with other grains
Arrowroot starch	A starchy thickener similar to cornstarch
Brown rice flour	Nutty flavor; gritty texture (unless milled superfine); more nutritious than white rice flour
Buckwheat flour	Strong, nutty flavor; high in protein; helps build structure in baked goods
Chickpea flour (garbanzo bean flour)	High in protein; sweet, beany taste; readily absorbs liquid and gets firm quickly; adds structure to gluten-free breads
Coconut flour	Rich in healthy fat; high in fiber; gently sweet coconut flavor; store in the refrigerator or freezer
Corn flour	Smooth and dense; mellow corn flavor
Cornmeal	Gritty texture; mild, sweet taste
Cornstarch	A smooth, excellent thickening starch
Flaxseed meal (ground flaxseeds)	Rich in fiber and antioxidants; can be used to replace eggs and add structure; store in the refrigerator or freezer
Garfava flour	A combination of chickpea flour and fava bean flour; has a slightly less beany taste than chickpea flour alone; store in the refrigerator or freezer
Millet flour	Sweet; easily digested; gritty unless ground superfine; store in the refrigerator or freezer
Potato flour	Heavy, white flour; adds density, smoothness, and a mild flavor to breads
Quinoa flour	Nutty, mild flavor; high in protein
Sorghum flour	Sweet, mild flavor; versatile
Soy flour	Nutty, sweet flavor; high in protein
Tapioca flour	Smooth, white flour; adds chewiness

Teff flour	Nutty tasting; nutrient dense
White rice flour	Bland tasting; gritty texture (unless milled superfine); combines well with other flours
Xanthan gum or guar gum	Gives a chewy mouthfeel to baked goods; xanthan gum is often preferred since guar gum can have a laxative effect

Grinding Your Own Gluten-Free Flours

It's easy to make a variety of gluten-free flours right in your own kitchen. You can use an electric grain grinder, which has blades designed specifically for this purpose, or you can use a sturdy, high-powered blender. Although most high-quality blenders can do a reasonable job of grinding grains in small quantities, using them regularly for this purpose can take a toll on their blades. Therefore, you might want to look into blenders that have blades and blender jars designed specifically for this purpose, such as a Blendtec kitchen mill or blender (blendtec.com), Vitamix blender (vitamix.com), or Breville Boss blender (brevilleusa.com). These powerful and versatile appliances can also grind spices and seasoning mixes, transform nuts and seeds into butters, and create purées, dips, and creamy desserts.

The appropriate machine can grind flours from gluten-free grains as well as from legumes (such as dried lentils and chickpeas), allowing you to make fresh gluten-free flours whenever you need them. It's much more cost-effective to grind your own flours, and doing so will provide you with a greater variety of gluten-free alternatives compared to what is available commercially. You will also be able to avoid the possibility of cross-contamination that can arise in a commercial mill where the same equipment may be used to grind wheat flours and gluten-free flours. For the best results and most even texture, sift home-ground flours after processing them.

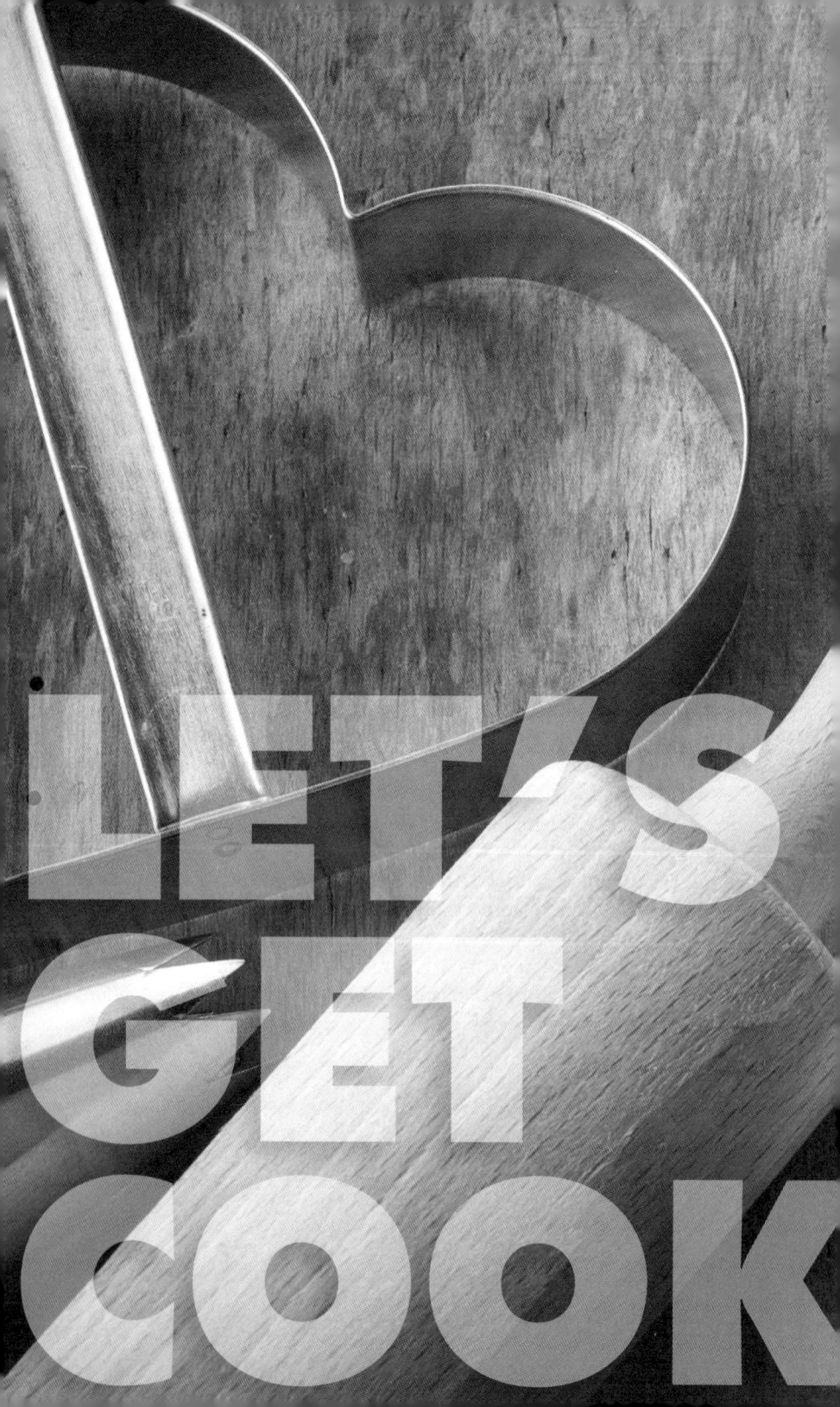

fundamentals

GF all-purpose flour mix

Use this incredibly adaptable, soy-free mix for both cooking and baking. Potato and arrowroot starches provide stickiness and adhesion, and chickpea and rice flours are sources of protein and iron. Combined, they provide a mix that is neutral in flavor and ideal to replace wheat flour in your favorite recipes.

> 3 cups potato starch or tapioca starch
> 2 cups chickpea flour
> 2 cups brown rice flour, white rice flour, or a combination
> 1 cup arrowroot starch

Put all the ingredients in a large bowl and whisk until well combined. Store in a sealed container at room temperature or in the refrigerator. Whisk or shake well before using in case any ingredients have settled.

TIPS

- When using this mix to replace wheat flour in conventional recipes, decrease the oven temperature by 25 degrees F and bake the item a little bit longer.

- When adapting conventional recipes for baked goods, add ¼ to ½ teaspoon of xanthan gum or ½ teaspoon of guar gum for each cup of flour called for in the recipe.

- Double the recipe if you want to keep a large amount on hand. The mix itself should not be frozen. However, chickpea flour and rice flour should be kept in the refrigerator or freezer for the longest storage. Potato starch and arrowroot should be stored in airtight containers at room temperature.

VARIATION: When using potato starch as the main ingredient, 1 cup of tapioca starch may be substituted for the arrowroot starch if desired.

Per ¼ cup: 136 calories, 2 g protein, 1 g fat (0 g sat), 31 g carbs, 1 mg sodium, 10 mg calcium, 2 g fiber

great gluten-free pizza crust

MAKES ONE 12-INCH REGULAR CRUST OR ONE 10-INCH THICK CRUST, 6 SERVINGS

Just because you can't have gluten doesn't mean you can't enjoy pizza! This crust holds together well and tastes delicious. In fact, it's so much quicker and tastier than yeasted, wheat-based pizza crust that even friends and family who are able to eat gluten will be clamoring for the recipe. Use any of your favorite toppings—sauce, veggies, gluten-free vegan cheese—and throw a pizza party!

1¾ cups GF All-Purpose Flour Mix (page 36) or other gluten-free all-purpose flour

¼ cup chickpea flour

¼ cup quinoa flour

1 teaspoon xanthan gum

½ teaspoon gluten-free baking powder

½ teaspoon sea salt

¼ cup extra-virgin olive oil

⅔ cup water

Preheat the oven to 425 degrees F. Generously oil one 12-inch or 10-inch pizza pan.

Put the flour mix, chickpea flour, quinoa flour, baking powder, and salt in a large bowl and whisk to combine. Stir in the oil using a fork, then work it in with your fingers. Pour in the water and stir until all the liquid is absorbed. The dough will be slightly sticky. Form into a ball.

Put the ball in the center of the oiled pizza pan and pat and press it into a disk, keeping the edges a little thicker to form a rim to contain the sauce and toppings. Patch any tears.

Bake for 10 minutes. Cool. Spread with your favorite sauce and toppings, then bake for 15 to 25 minutes (depending on the thickness of the crust), or until the edges are golden brown.

Per serving: 277 calories, 4 g protein, 11 g fat (1 g sat), 42 g carbs, 160 mg sodium, 21 mg calcium, 4 g fiber

perfection pie crust

This recipe is super easy to make and the dough is very forgiving. The taste is delicious, and the texture is light, crispy, and flaky. Double the recipe to make a top crust or to make two pies.

> 1 cup GF All-Purpose Flour Mix (page 36) or other gluten-free all-purpose flour, plus more as needed
>
> 2 tablespoons quinoa flour
>
> ½ teaspoon xanthan gum
>
> ¼ teaspoon sea salt
>
> 6 tablespoons vegetable shortening or coconut oil
>
> 3 tablespoons cold water, plus more as needed

Put the flour mix, quinoa flour, xanthan gum, and salt in a large bowl. Cut in the shortening using a pastry blender, a fork, or two knives until the particles are the size of small peas. Sprinkle the water over the flour mixture. Toss and stir with a fork until the mixture starts to cling and a ball can be formed. If the dough appears too dry, add up to 1 tablespoon of additional cold water, 1 teaspoon at a time, mixing well after each addition. If the dough is too sticky, sprinkle a bit more flour mix over it.

Lightly sprinkle a flat surface with additional flour mix. Turn the dough out of the bowl onto the floured surface and gently knead 6 to 10 times to form a ball. Moisten a clean area of the work surface with water. Tear off a 12-inch piece of waxed paper and put it on the moist surface. Put the dough on the waxed paper and top with another piece of waxed paper. Roll out the crust between the two sheets of waxed paper into a 10- to 12-inch disk. (The moist work surface will help keep the waxed paper from sliding around.)

Remove and discard the top piece of waxed paper. Slip your hand under the bottom sheet of waxed paper and gently flip the dough over a 9-inch pie plate, carefully easing it in with the waxed paper that's now on top. Use the waxed paper to help press the dough gently against the sides and bottom of the pie pan. Carefully remove the waxed paper. Flute the edges, fill with your choice of fillings, and bake according to your favorite pie-recipe directions. If using a top crust, vent it and trim the edges before fluting.

For a prebaked shell (to use with cooked pudding or any other filling that doesn't require further baking), preheat the oven to 400 degrees F. Prick the bottom and sides of the crust with a fork and bake for 20 minutes. Cool completely before filling.

Per serving: 159 calories, 1 g protein, 9 g fat (2 g sat), 17 g carbs, 57 mg sodium, 5 mg calcium, 1 g fiber

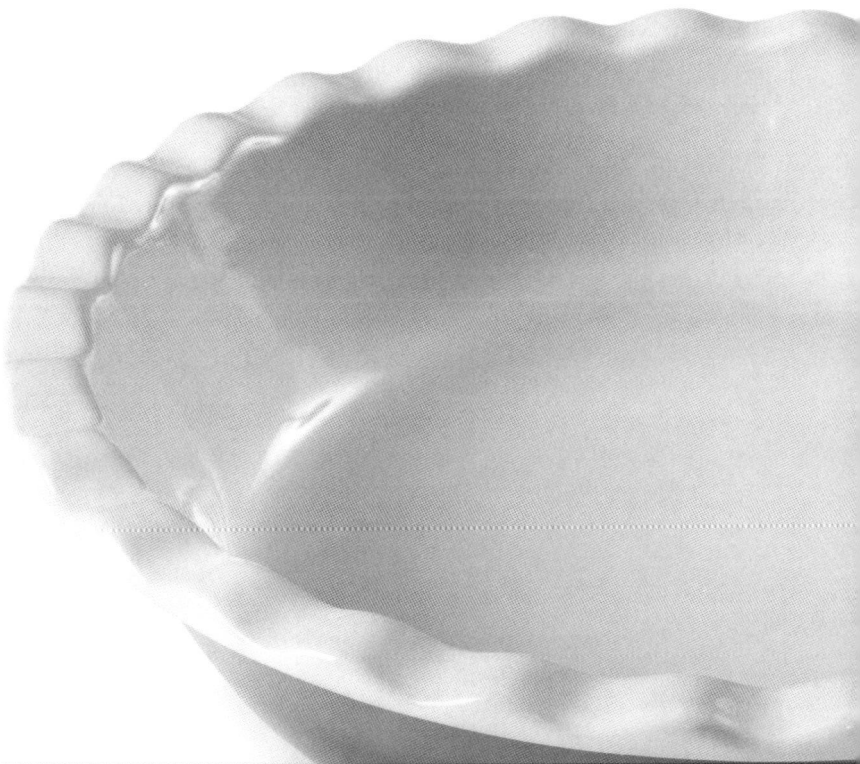

pat-in-the-pan pie crust

This amazing crust is exceptionally rich and flaky—perfect for all your sweet or savory pies.

> 2 cups GF All-Purpose Flour Mix (page 36) or other gluten-free all-purpose flour
>
> 2 teaspoons unbleached cane sugar or coconut sugar
>
> 1 teaspoon sea salt
>
> 1 teaspoon xanthan gum
>
> 6 tablespoons soft coconut oil
>
> ⅓ cup water
>
> 2 tablespoons extra-virgin olive oil

Put the flour mix, sugar, salt, and xanthan gum in a 9- or 10-inch pie pan. Stir with a fork to combine. Add the coconut oil, water, and olive oil and stir with the fork to combine. Finish by using your fingers. Pat and press the crust into the bottom of the pie pan and up the sides. Prick the bottom and sides all over with the tines of a fork and flute the edges.

Fill with your favorite filling and bake as directed in the recipe. For a prebaked shell (to use with cooked pudding or any other filling that doesn't require further baking), preheat the oven to 400 degrees F. Prick the bottom and sides of the crust with a fork and bake for 25 minutes. Cool completely before filling.

Per serving: 259 calories, 2 g protein, 15 g fat (10 g sat), 32 g carbs, 224 mg sodium, 10 mg calcium, 2 g fiber

gomasio

Sesame seeds and sea vegetables, such as kelp, dulse, and nori, are rich in minerals. Sprinkled over vegetables, soups, grains, or beans, gomasio will deepen the overall flavor of any dish.

½ cup hulled sesame seeds
½ teaspoon sea salt
¼ teaspoon kelp, dulse, or nori powder

Dry-roast the sesame seeds in a skillet over medium heat, stirring frequently, until the seeds can be crushed between your thumb and finger, 5 to 7 minutes. Transfer to a mortar or mini food processor. Add the salt and kelp powder. Using the pestle and grinding in a circular motion, or using pulse action of the processor, grind the seeds until about two-thirds of them are crushed and coated with their own oil. Stored in a sealed jar in the refrigerator, gomasio will keep for 4 weeks.

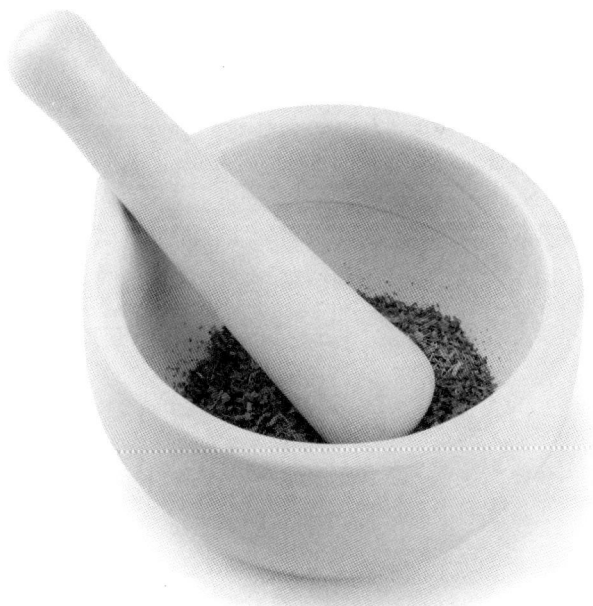

Per 1 tablespoon: 53 calories, 2 g protein, 5 g fat (1 g sat), 2 g carbs, 126 mg sodium, 15 mg calcium, 1 g fiber

garam masala

This popular Indian blend of sweet spices is warming rather than hot. It's traditionally used to flavor rice or bean dishes and even desserts.

- 4 teaspoons ground coriander
- 2 teaspoons ground cumin
- 1 teaspoon freshly ground black pepper
- 1 teaspoon ground cinnamon
- 1 teaspoon ground cloves

Put all the ingredients in a small jar, seal tightly, and shake well to combine.

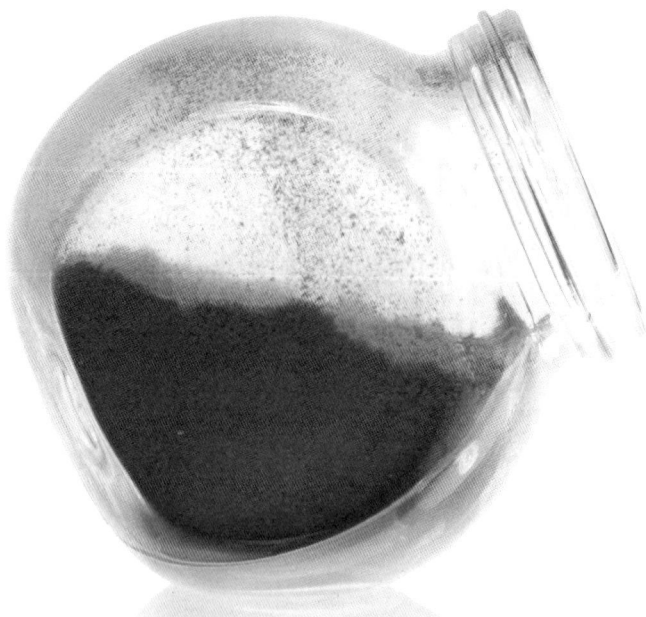

Per 1 teaspoon: 8 calories, 0 g protein, 0 g fat (0 g sat), 1 g carbs, 2 mg sodium, 13 mg calcium, 1 g fiber

creole spice blend

Add a blast of the bayou to your favorite soups, stews, and sauces. Filé powder (also called gumbo filé) is made from the ground dried leaves of the sassafras tree. Its woodsy flavor is reminiscent of root beer. Filé powder is integral to Creole cuisine and is used to thicken and flavor gumbos and other Creole dishes. This spice mixture is best stirred into a dish after it has finished cooking because too much heat can make filé tough and stringy. Look for filé powder in the spice or gourmet section of your supermarket.

2 tablespoons paprika
2 tablespoons dried basil
2 tablespoons dried thyme
1 tablespoon cayenne
1 tablespoon filé powder
1½ teaspoons gluten-free chili powder

Put all the ingredients in asmall jar, seal tightly, and shake well to combine.

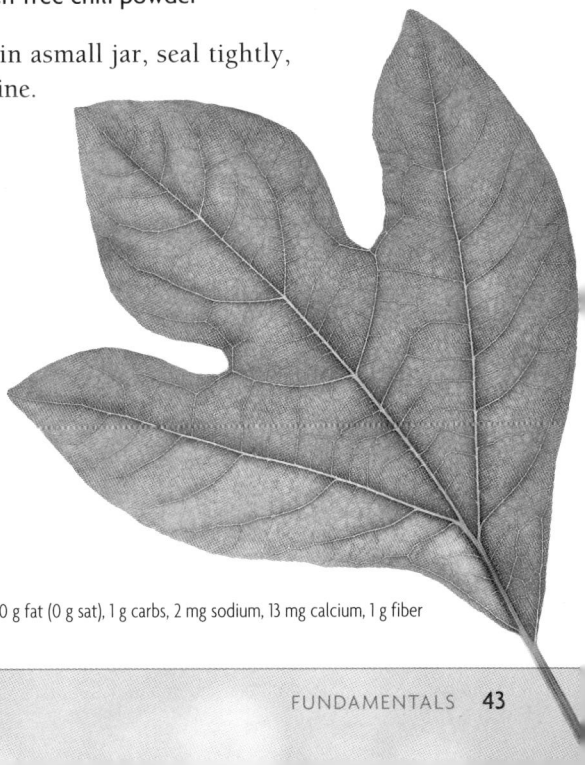

Per 1 teaspoon: 8 calories, 0 g protein, 0 g fat (0 g sat), 1 g carbs, 2 mg sodium, 13 mg calcium, 1 g fiber

kick-it-up spice blend

MAKES ⅔ CUP

Use a pinch of this mix whenever you want to kick up the flavor of your food several notches. It's spicy, so add it gradually.

2½ tablespoons paprika
2 tablespoons sea salt
2 tablespoons garlic powder
1 tablespoon freshly ground black pepper
1 tablespoon cayenne
1 tablespoon onion powder
1 tablespoon dried oregano
1 tablespoon dried thyme

Put all the ingredients in a small jar, seal tightly, and shake well to combine.

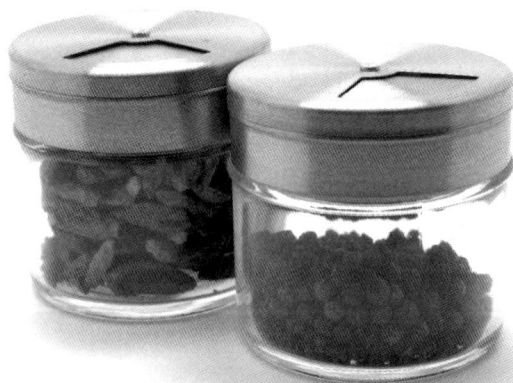

Per 1 teaspoon: 6 calories, 0 g protein, 0 g fat (0 g sat), 1 g carbs, 331 mg sodium, 7 mg calcium, 1 g fiber

five-alarm chili powder

This chili powder is more intense and pungent than packaged brands, so you might need to use a little less than usual. Some commercial brands contain gluten, but making chili powder from scratch is easy, and you'll know exactly what is—and isn't—in it.

6 tablespoons paprika

2 tablespoons ground turmeric

1 tablespoon crushed red chile flakes

1 teaspoon ground cumin

1 teaspoon dried oregano

½ teaspoon cayenne

½ teaspoon garlic powder

½ teaspoon sea salt

¼ teaspoon ground cloves

Put all the ingredients in a food processor and grind into a fine powder. Alternatively, grind the chile flakes into a fine powder and combine them in a jar with the remaining ingredients. Seal tightly and shake well until evenly combined.

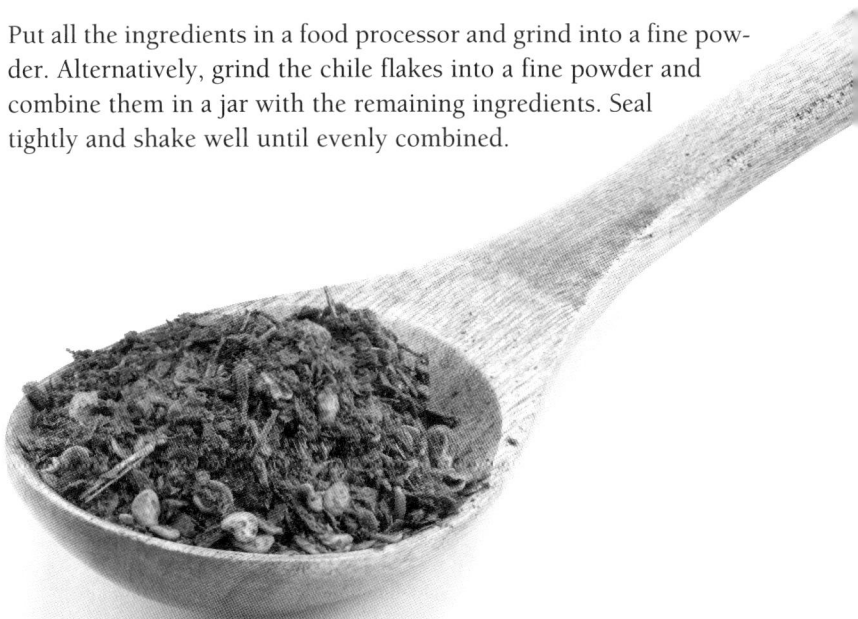

Per 1 teaspoon: 8 calories, 0 g protein, 0 g fat (0 g sat), 1 g carbs, 38 mg sodium, 7 mg calcium, 1 g fiber

all-purpose herb blend

Use this tasty, salt-free, gluten-free, all-purpose herbal mix to heighten the flavor of soups, salads, dressings, grains, and vegetables.

1 tablespoon dried thyme

1 tablespoon dried oregano

2 teaspoons rubbed sage

1 teaspoon dried basil

1 teaspoon dried marjoram

1 teaspoon dried parsley flakes

1 teaspoon dried rosemary

Put all the ingredients in a small jar, seal tightly, and shake well to combine.

Per 1 teaspoon: 3 calories, 0 g protein, 0 g fat (0 g sat), 1 g carbs, 1 mg sodium, 19 mg calcium, 1 g fiber

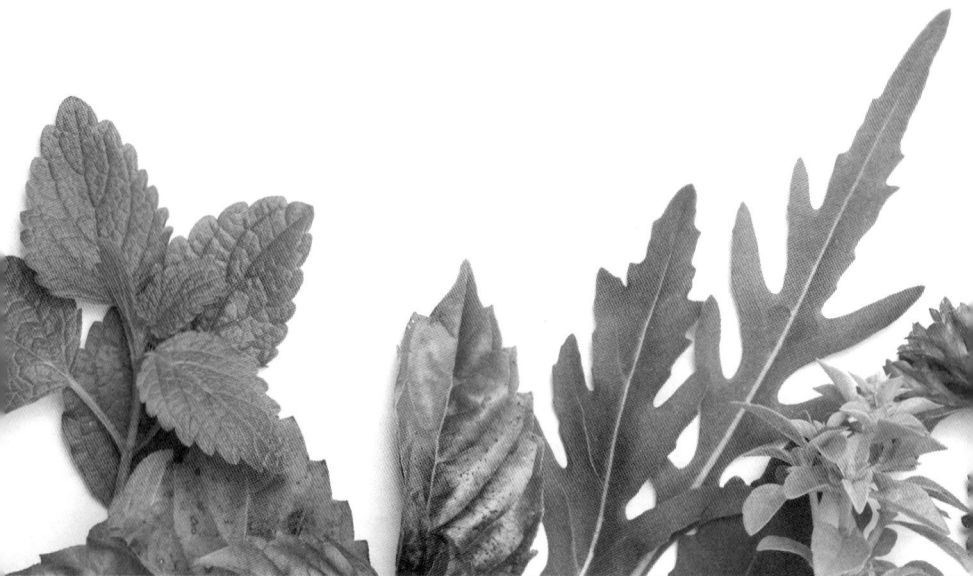

italian seasoning

MAKES 1 CUP

Punch up the flavor of your tomato sauce, Italian dressing, and other Italian specialties with this simple and fragrant herbal blend. If you prefer a powder, just buzz everything in a food processor or blender until finely ground.

¼ cup dried basil
¼ cup dried parsley
2 tablespoons dried minced garlic
2 tablespoons dried minced onion
2 tablespoons dried oregano
1 tablespoon dried thyme
1 teaspoon freshly ground black pepper
¼ teaspoon rubbed sage

Put all the ingredients in a small jar, seal tightly, and shake well to combine.

Per 1 teaspoon: 3 calories, 0 g protein, 0 g fat (0 g sat), 1 g carbs, 1 mg sodium, 23 mg calcium, 1 g fiber

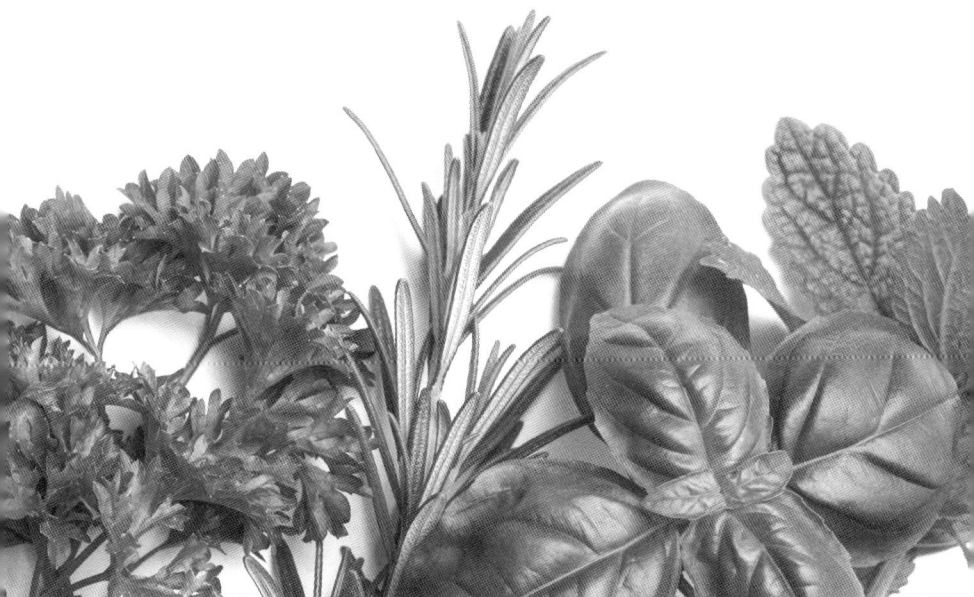

ethiopian spice mix

This simple twist on Ethiopian berbere is a snappy mix that will turn up the heat and flavor of any soup, stew, vegetable, or bean dish. Start with a small amount and add more gradually as you see fit.

2 tablespoons paprika

1½ tablespoons cayenne

1 tablespoon onion powder (optional)

1 teaspoon garlic powder (optional)

1 teaspoon dried basil

½ teaspoon ground ginger

¼ teaspoon ground allspice

¼ teaspoon ground cardamom

¼ teaspoon ground cinnamon

¼ teaspoon ground cumin

¼ teaspoon ground fenugreek

¼ teaspoon ground nutmeg

¼ teaspoon freshly ground black pepper

¼ teaspoon ground turmeric

⅛ teaspoon ground cloves

Put all the ingredients in a small jar, seal tightly, and shake well to combine.

Per 1 teaspoon: 7 calories, 0 g protein, 0 g fat (0 g sat), 2 g carbs, 1 mg sodium, 8 mg calcium, 1 g fiber

sweet-and-hot mix

MAKES ½ CUP

This aromatic blend combines both sweet and hot Indian spices. It adds spark and tang to tomato and potato dishes and is especially delicious as a soup or vegetable seasoning. It's extremely hot, however, so use with caution.

1 tablespoon cayenne
1 tablespoon ground cumin
1 tablespoon ground coriander
1½ teaspoons ground fenugreek
1 teaspoon ground cardamom
1 teaspoon ground cinnamon
1 teaspoon ground cloves
1 teaspoon ground nutmeg
¼ teaspoon sea salt
¼ teaspoon freshly ground black pepper
¼ teaspoon ground turmeric

Put all the ingredients in a small jar, seal tightly, and shake well to combine.

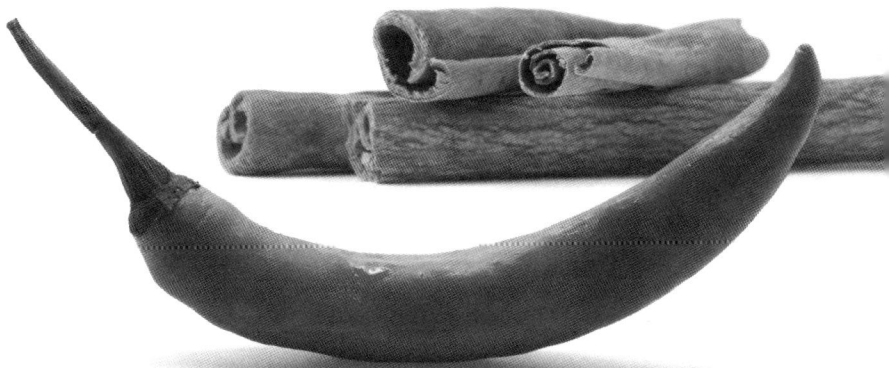

Per 1 teaspoon: 3 calories, 0 g protein, 0 g fat (0 g sat), 1 g carbs, 20 mg sodium, 7 mg calcium, 0 g fiber

bread basket

sunny seed bread

This bread is delicious for breakfast, snacks, or sandwiches. It's not too sweet, which makes it quite versatile, and every single bite packs a delightful crunch.

2 cups GF All-Purpose Flour Mix (page 36) or other gluten-free all-purpose flour

1 tablespoon gluten-free baking powder

1 teaspoon xanthan gum

½ teaspoon sea salt

⅓ cup raw sunflower seeds

2 tablespoons raw or toasted sesame seeds or raw pumpkin seeds

2 tablespoons poppy seeds (optional)

2 tablespoons tahini or sunflower seed butter

1 cup water, gluten-free plain or vanilla nondairy milk, or lite coconut milk

⅓ cup melted coconut oil

⅓ cup pure maple syrup

1 teaspoon cider vinegar or freshly squeezed lemon juice

Preheat the oven to 350 degrees F. Generously oil a metal 8½ x 4½ x 2½-inch loaf pan.

Combine the flour mix, baking powder, xanthan gum, and salt in a large bowl and whisk until well combined. Stir in the sunflower seeds, sesame seeds, and optional poppy seeds.

Put the tahini in a small bowl. Gradually whisk in the water, beating vigorously until smooth and milky. Whisk in the oil, maple syrup, and vinegar until well combined. Pour into the dry ingredients and stir until just combined. Spoon into the oiled loaf pan and smooth the top with a silicone spatula.

Bake for 60 to 70 minutes, or until a toothpick inserted in the center tests clean. Let cool in the pan on a rack for 10 minutes. Remove from the pan and let cool completely on the rack before slicing or storing.

Per slice: 231 calories, 1 g protein, 12 g fat (6 g sat), 28 g carbs, 93 mg sodium, 40 mg calcium, 1 g fiber

magical one-bowl muffins

Although these gluten-free muffins are "plain," they're mighty tasty, especially when served with jam or fruit butter. Their magic comes into play with all the variations that are possible, from sweet to savory.

> 2 cups GF All-Purpose Flour Mix (page 36) or other gluten-free all-purpose flour
>
> ½ cup unbleached cane sugar
>
> 1 tablespoon gluten-free baking powder
>
> ½ teaspoon sea salt
>
> ½ teaspoon xanthan gum
>
> 2 cups gluten-free nondairy milk or water
>
> ½ cup melted coconut oil or other neutral oil

Preheat the oven to 375 degrees F. Line a twelve-cup standard muffin pan with baking cups.

Put the flour mix, sugar, baking powder, salt, and xanthan gum in a medium bowl and whisk until well combined. Add the milk and oil and whisk until smooth and well combined. Spoon equally into the baking cups (do not overfill). Bake on the center rack for 25 minutes, until lightly browned and a toothpick inserted in the center of a muffin tests clean. Turn out onto a rack to cool. The muffins are best served warm.

Per muffin: 192 calories, 1 g protein, 11 g fat (8 g sat), 23 g carbs, 112 mg sodium, 44 mg calcium, 0 g fiber
Note: Analysis is for the basic recipe only.

TIPS

- If you choose not to use baking cups to line the muffin pan, be sure to generously oil the pan. Baking cups are strongly recommended, however. They will not only make cleanup much easier, they will help keep the muffins soft, tender, and moist.
- Additions such as seeds, nuts, raisins, or more sweetener will increase the amount of batter, and you may need to prepare an additional muffin cup or two to accommodate the larger quantity.

BLANK-SLATE QUICK BREAD: Preheat the oven to 350 degrees F. Generously oil a metal 9 x 5-inch loaf pan. Use any of the variations that follow. Pour into the prepared loaf pan and bake on the center rack for 60 to 70 minutes, or until a toothpick inserted in the center tests clean.

CHOCOLATE MUFFINS: Increase the sugar to ¾ cup and add 3 tablespoons of unsweetened gluten-free cocoa powder to the dry ingredients.

CINNAMON-RAISIN MUFFINS: Add ½ teaspoon of ground cinnamon to the dry ingredients. Add ½ cup of raisins to the batter just before spooning into the muffin cups.

CRUNCHY SEED OR NUT MUFFINS: Stir ¼ cup of sesame or sunflower seeds or ½ cup of chopped walnuts, pecans, almonds, or cashews into the batter. Roasting the seeds or nuts first will give them a deeper, richer flavor.

DILLY MUFFINS: Add 2 teaspoons of dried dill weed to the dry ingredients.

DRIED FRUIT MUFFINS: Add ½ cup of raisins, chopped dates, or chopped dried apricots to the batter just before spooning into the muffin cups.

LEMON–POPPY SEED MUFFINS: Add ¼ cup of poppy seeds to the dry ingredients and add 1 teaspoon of gluten-free lemon extract when whisking in the milk.

MAPLE CORN MUFFINS: Replace 1½ cups of the flour mix with yellow or blue cornmeal. Omit the sugar and combine ½ cup of maple syrup with the milk and oil.

MARMALADE MUFFINS: Omit the sugar. Combine the water and oil with ½ cup of orange marmalade.

ONION-HERB MUFFINS: Decrease the sugar to 2 teaspoons and add 1 teaspoon of dried thyme and 1 teaspoon of dried rosemary to the dry ingredients. Stir ½ cup of finely chopped onions into the batter just before spooning into the muffin cups.

ORANGE MUFFINS: Replace 1 cup of the milk with 1 cup of orange juice and add ½ teaspoon of gluten-free orange extract.

QUINOA-CORN MUFFINS: Replace 1½ cups of the flour mix with 1½ cups of yellow cornmeal and 1 tablespoon of quinoa flour.

pumpkin spice bread

This delicious bread, with its perfect balance of sweetness and spice, is ideal on crisp fall mornings. The heavenly aroma will make your whole house smell fantastic.

¾ cup canned pumpkin purée

½ cup light brown sugar, firmly packed

½ cup pure maple syrup

⅓ cup organic canola, safflower, or other neutral oil

¼ cup applesauce

1½ cups GF All-Purpose Flour Mix (page 36) or other gluten-free all-purpose flour

¼ cup quinoa flour

1½ teaspoons gluten-free baking powder

1½ teaspoons baking soda

1 teaspoon ground cinnamon

1 teaspoon xanthan gum

½ teaspoon ground allspice

½ teaspoon sea salt

¼ teaspoon ground cloves

¼ teaspoon ground ginger

¼ teaspoon ground nutmeg

½ cup chopped pecans (optional)

½ cup raisins, dried cherries, or currants (optional)

Preheat the oven to 350 degrees F. Generously oil a metal 8½ x 4½ x 2½-inch loaf pan.

Put the pumpkin, brown sugar, maple syrup, oil, and applesauce in large bowl. Beat with an electric mixer on low speed until very smooth, about 1 minute.

Put the flour mix, quinoa flour, baking powder, baking soda, cinnamon, xanthan gum, allspice, salt, cloves, ginger, and nutmeg in a separate large bowl and whisk until well combined. Gradually beat the dry ingredients into the pumpkin mixture in three additions with the mixer on low speed. Stir in the pecans and raisins if using.

Pour into the oiled loaf pan and smooth out the top with a silicone spatula. Bake for 60 to 70 minutes, or until a toothpick inserted in the center tests clean.

Cool in the pan on a wire rack for 10 minutes. Remove the bread from the pan and cool upside down on the rack for 20 to 30 minutes. Turn upright and cool completely before slicing. Tightly wrapped, the bread will keep for 2 days at room temperature or for 3 days in the refrigerator.

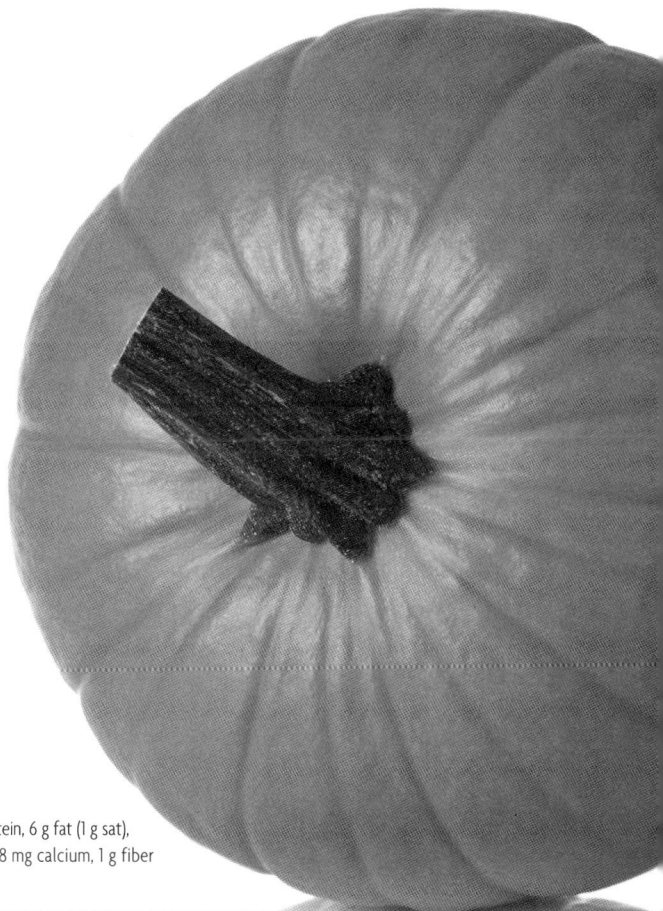

Per slice: 184 calories, 2 g protein, 6 g fat (1 g sat), 20 g carbs, 234 mg sodium, 18 mg calcium, 1 g fiber

banana bread

Moist and flavorful banana bread makes a tasty breakfast or nutritious snack. It's a great way to use up bananas that are getting a tad too ripe.

¾ cup light brown sugar, firmly packed

¼ cup organic canola oil, safflower oil, or other neutral oil

1 teaspoon gluten-free vanilla extract

1¾ cups GF All-Purpose Flour Mix (page 36) or other gluten-free all-purpose flour

2 teaspoons gluten-free baking powder

1¼ teaspoons ground cinnamon

1 teaspoon xanthan gum

½ teaspoon sea salt

1½ cups mashed ripe bananas (about 3 medium)

½ cup chopped walnuts or pecans (optional)

½ cup raisins or dark chocolate chips (optional)

Preheat the oven to 350 degrees F. Generously oil a metal 8½ x 4½ x 2½-inch loaf pan.

Put the brown sugar, oil, and vanilla extract in a large bowl and stir until well combined. Put the flour mix, baking powder, cinnamon, xanthan gum, and salt in a medium bowl and whisk until well combined. Stir the flour mixture into the wet ingredients in three additions, alternating with the mashed bananas and ending with the flour mixture. Stir in the walnuts and raisins if using. The batter will be somewhat soft. Pour into the oiled loaf pan.

Bake for 60 to 70 minutes, or until a toothpick inserted in the center tests clean. Cool in the pan on a wire rack for 10 minutes. Remove from the pan and cool upside down on the rack for 20 to 30 minutes. Turn upright and cool completely before slicing. Tightly wrapped, the bread will keep for 2 days at room temperature or for 3 days in the refrigerator.

Per slice: 160 calories, 1 g protein, 5 g fat (1 g sat), 28 g carbs, 84 mg sodium, 12 mg calcium, 1 g fiber

vanilla-currant scones

Scones are tender, lightly sweetened, biscuit-like cakes. Serve them with jam or gluten-free vegan butter or both. They tend to dry out quickly but will remain soft for a few days if stored in a sealed container with a wedge of apple, which adds moisture.

> 2¾ cups GF All-Purpose Flour Mix (page 36) or other gluten-free all-purpose flour
> ¼ cup unbleached cane sugar
> 2 teaspoons gluten-free baking powder
> ½ teaspoon xanthan gum
> ¼ teaspoon sea salt
> ⅓ cup soft coconut oil
> ½ cup water
> ¼ cup pure maple syrup
> 2 tablespoons applesauce
> 1 tablespoon gluten-free vanilla extract
> ⅓ cup dried currants or raisins

Preheat the oven to 400 degrees F. Line a baking sheet with parchment paper or a silicone baking mat.

Put the flour mix, sugar, baking powder, xanthan gum, and salt in a large bowl and whisk until well combined. Stir in the oil using a fork, then work it in with your fingers until the mixture resembles fine crumbs.

Put the water, maple syrup, applesauce, and vanilla extract in a small bowl and stir to combine. Pour into the dry ingredients and stir until evenly combined. Add the currants and knead in the bowl until evenly distributed, about 30 seconds.

Put the dough on the lined baking sheet and pat it into an 8-inch disk. Cut it into 12 equal wedges using a sharp knife and carefully separate the wedges so they have room to expand. If the knife becomes sticky, rinse it off. Bake the scones for 20 to 25 minutes, until the edges are lightly golden. Remove from the oven and put the baking sheet on a wire rack. Let the scones cool on the pan for 5 minutes, then transfer them to the rack to finish cooling. The scones are best served warm.

Per scone: 216 calories, 2 g protein, 6 g fat (5 g sat), 38 g carbs, 49 mg sodium, 20 mg calcium, 2 g fiber

gluten-free chapatis

Native to India, chapatis are round, flat, unleavened breads cooked on a griddle. Although chapatis are traditionally made with wheat, you'll find this gluten-free version to be equally as versatile, tender, and tasty. Chapatis make a great accompaniment to dips, soups, and stews instead of bread, crackers, or rolls. You can also gently fold a chapati in half like a soft-shell taco and fill it with seasoned beans, or use it like a thick slice of bread to make a sandwich.

2 cups GF All-Purpose Flour Mix (page 36) or other gluten-free all-purpose flour, plus more as needed

1 teaspoon gluten-free baking powder

1 teaspoon sea salt

½ teaspoon unbleached cane sugar

¼ teaspoon xanthan gum

2 tablespoons soft coconut oil

¾ cup warm water, plus more as needed

Put the flour mix, baking powder, salt, sugar, and xanthan gum in a large bowl and whisk until well combined. Cut in the coconut oil using a pastry blender, a fork, or two knives, then finish working it in with your hands. Add the warm water, starting with ¾ cup. Mix well using a fork and then your hands. Continue to add water as needed until a soft, cohesive dough is formed. If the dough is dry, add up to 4 tablespoons of additional water as needed, adding 1 tablespoon at a time; if the dough is sticky, add a little extra flour mix.

Lightly sprinkle a flat surface with additional flour mix. Transfer the dough to the floured surface and knead for 5 minutes. Return the dough to the bowl, cover with plastic wrap, and let rest for 30 minutes.

Heat a nonstick griddle or nonstick skillet over medium heat. Moisten a clean area of the work surface with water. Tear off a 12-inch piece of waxed paper and put it on the moist surface.

While the griddle is heating, divide the dough into six equal pieces. Work with one piece at a time and cover the remaining pieces so they don't dry out. Put the dough on the waxed paper and top with another piece of waxed paper. Roll the dough between the two sheets of waxed paper into a disk about ⅛ inch thick and 6 to 8 inches in diameter. Carefully peel off the top sheet of waxed paper and flip the chapati over so it is resting in your open palm and the remaining sheet of waxed paper is now on top. Carefully remove the remaining sheet of waxed paper and gently flip the chapati onto the hot griddle.

Cook one chapati at a time until lightly puffed, the surface has a few bubbles, and the bottom has a few brown flecks, 1 to 2 minutes. Turn it over and cook the second side briefly, just until lightly browned, about 1 minute. Keep the cooked chapatis wrapped in a clean tea towel until ready to serve. This will keep them warm, soft, and pliable.

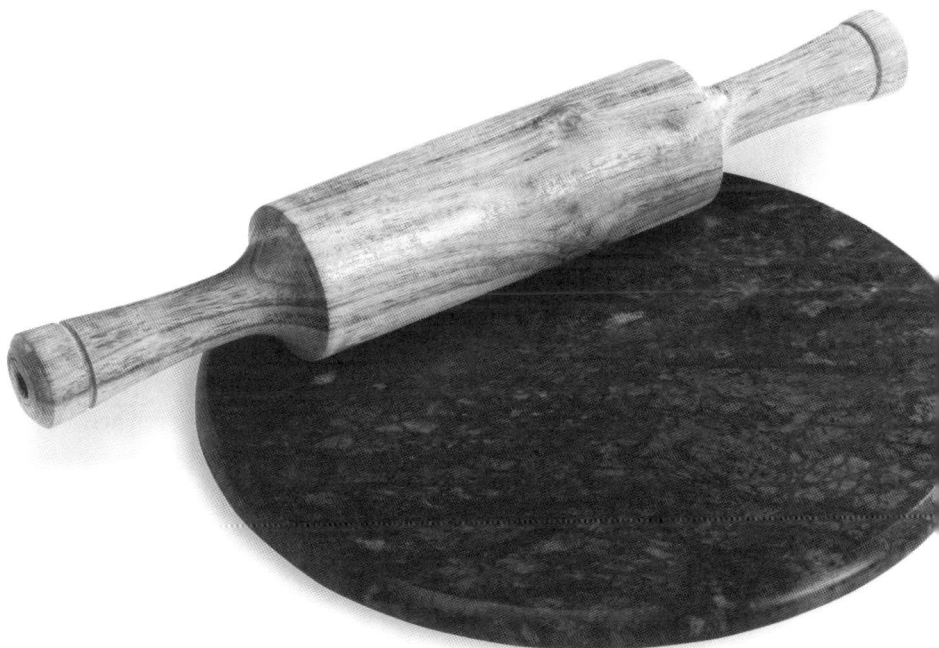

Per chapati: 222 calories, 3 g protein, 6 g fat (4 g sat), 41 g carbs, 304 mg sodium, 13 mg calcium, 5 g fiber

cornbread squares

These versatile squares have just a hint of sweetness, which makes them great to serve with either savory or sweet dishes. Try them for breakfast slathered with fruit spread or coconut butter, or partner them with gluten-free vegan chili and a garden-fresh salad for dinner.

1½ cups yellow cornmeal

½ cup GF All-Purpose Flour Mix (page 36) or other gluten-free all-purpose flour

1 tablespoon gluten-free baking powder

½ teaspoon sea salt

½ teaspoon xanthan gum

1 cup water

½ cup pure maple syrup

½ cup melted coconut oil

Preheat the oven to 350 degrees F. Generously oil an 8-inch square metal baking pan.

Put the cornmeal, flour mix, baking powder, salt, and xanthan gum in a large bowl and whisk until well combined.

Put the water, maple syrup, and oil in a small bowl and stir to combine. Pour into the flour mixture and whisk vigorously until well combined and nearly lump-free. Pour into the oiled baking pan, using a silicone spatula to scrape out the bowl. Bake on the center rack of the oven for 45 to 50 minutes, or until a toothpick inserted in the center tests clean.

Put the pan on a wire rack and let the cornbread cool completely in the pan before cutting. Tightly wrapped, the cornbread will keep for 2 days at room temperature or for 3 days in the refrigerator.

Per square: 257 calories, 2 g protein, 13 g fat (11 g sat), 35 g carbs, 128 mg sodium, 21 mg calcium, 2 g fiber

chickpea crêpes

Use these savory crêpes to complement any grain or vegetable dish or load them with your favorite fillings and roll them up like tortillas.

>   1 cup chickpea flour
>   ¼ teaspoon garlic powder (optional)
>   ¼ teaspoon ground turmeric
>   ¼ teaspoon sea salt
>   1 cup water

Put the flour in a large, dry skillet and cook, stirring almost constantly, over medium heat until it turns a shade darker, emits a nutty aroma, and no longer tastes raw, about 5 minutes. Transfer to a medium bowl and stir in the optional garlic powder, turmeric, and salt. Gradually whisk in the water, beating vigorously until the mixture is lump-free and completely smooth.

Oil a small, heavy skillet (preferably nonstick) with coconut oil and heat over medium-high heat. When the skillet is hot, drop a scant ¼ cup of the batter into it and immediately rotate the skillet to spread the batter evenly and make a thin round. Cook until the crêpe begins to brown on the bottom, 1 to 2 minutes. (The cooking time will depend on how hot the skillet is and how thick the crêpe is.) Carefully turn the crêpe over and cook the other side until lightly brown, about 1 minute. Repeat until all the batter is used up, adding more oil to the pan between each crêpe.

Stack the crêpes on a plate or clean tea towel after they are cooked. Cover them with a clean tea towel to keep them warm and soft until serving time.

Per crepe: 59 calories, 3 g protein, 1 g fat (0 g sat), 9 g carbs, 83 mg sodium, 0 mg calcium, 2 g fiber

silver dollar pancakes

The trick to good pancakes is to preheat the skillet so a drop of water dances across the surface. Serve these scrumptious mini pancakes with pure maple syrup and gluten-free vegan butter or your favorite pancake toppings.

½ cup brown rice flour

½ cup chickpea flour

1½ teaspoons gluten-free baking powder

¾ cup gluten-free plain or vanilla nondairy milk

1 tablespoon soft coconut oil, safflower oil, or other neutral oil, plus more for cooking

½ cup fresh blueberries (optional)

Put the rice flour, chickpea flour, and baking powder in a medium bowl and whisk until well combined. Put the milk and oil in a small bowl or measuring cup and stir to combine. Pour into the flour mixture and whisk until smooth and lump-free. Stir in the blueberries if using.

Oil a large, heavy skillet or griddle (preferably nonstick) with coconut oil and heat over medium-high heat. When hot, spoon in the batter using about 1 tablespoon to make each 2-inch pancake. Cook the pancakes until lightly browned and bubbles pop through the top, 1 to 2 minutes. Turn over and cook the other side until lightly browned, about 1 minute. To prevent sticking, oil the skillet well between batches.

Per pancake: 36 calories, 1 g protein, 1 g fat (1 g sat), 5 g carbs, 14 mg sodium, 21 mg calcium, 1 g fiber
Note: Analysis doesn't include additional coconut oil for cooking.

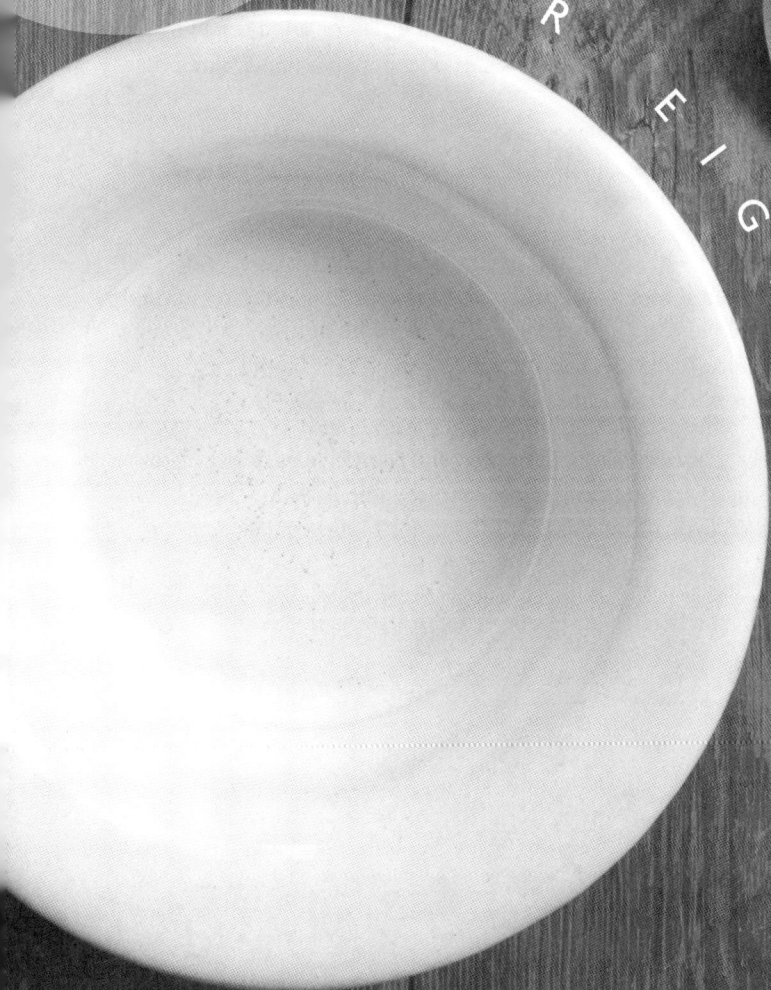

breakfast bowl

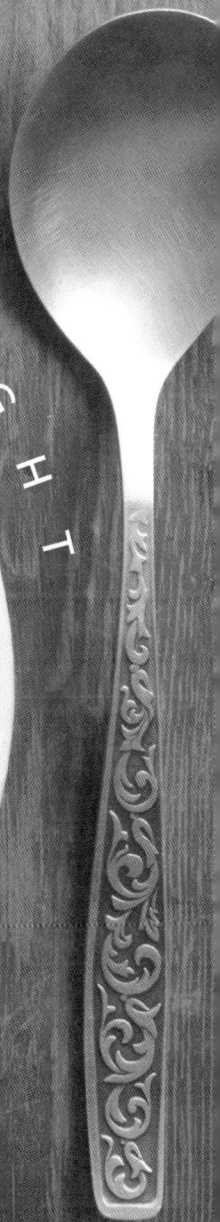

good morning muesli

This creamy, nourishing breakfast can be prepared with ease the night before, and leftovers make a delicious evening snack. It's also great to take on camping trips or when traveling. Just make it in advance and store it in spill-proof containers.

¾ cup rolled brown rice flakes (see tip), quinoa flakes, or a combination

2 tablespoons raisins, currants, dried cherries, or dried cranberries

2 tablespoons raw sunflower seeds or chopped walnuts, almonds, or pecans (optional)

¼ teaspoon ground cinnamon

1 cup gluten-free plain or vanilla nondairy milk or fruit juice, plus more as needed

1 apple, finely chopped (peeling optional)

Put the rice flakes, raisins, optional sunflower seeds, and cinnamon in a medium bowl and stir to combine. Add the milk and stir to combine. Cover and refrigerate for 8 to 12 hours. Stir in the apple just before serving. Serve with additional milk if desired.

TIP: Rolled brown rice flakes are roasted and rolled flakes of rice. They're similar to rolled oats and can be used in the same fashion. One popular brand of rolled brown rice flakes is Eden Foods (edenfoods.com/store).

VARIATION: Replace the apple with a banana, mango, nectarine, peach, or mango, or use berries or whatever fresh fruit is in season.

Per serving: 338 calories, 5 g protein, 7 g fat (0.4 g sat), 67 g carbs, 82 mg sodium, 247 mg calcium, 5 g fiber

amaranth, quinoa, and polenta porridge

MAKES 4 SERVINGS

This delightful combination of whole grains makes for a low-fat, protein-packed breakfast that will fill you up without weighing you down. Although this recipe makes a good quantity, leftovers keep well and reheat beautifully.

CEREAL

⅓ cup amaranth

⅓ cup quinoa

⅓ cup yellow corn grits (polenta)

Pinch ground cinnamon (optional)

Pinch sea salt

3½ cups water

OPTIONAL TOPPINGS

Berries

Fresh fruit, chopped

Raw or toasted nuts, chopped, or seeds

Gluten-free plain or vanilla nondairy milk

Gluten-free vegan butter

Pure maple syrup

Put the amaranth, quinoa, grits, optional cinnamon, and salt in a medium saucepan. Add the water and bring to a boil over medium-high heat. Decrease the heat to low and simmer uncovered, stirring frequently, until most of the water is absorbed and the grains are tender, about 25 minutes. Serve immediately with the toppings of your choice.

TIP: Stored in a sealed container in the refrigerator, leftover porridge will keep for 2 days. The porridge will thicken when chilled. Reheat on the stove or in a microwave, adding additional water or milk to achieve the desired consistency.

Per serving: 338 calories, 11 g protein, 6 g fat (1 g sat), 62 g carbs, 21 mg sodium, 111 mg calcium, 6 g fiber

Note: Analysis does not include optional toppings.

creamy golden porridge

The Aztecs believed amaranth had special properties that would give them amazing strength. Because of this, it became one of the main foods of the Aztec royalty. This tasty, power-packed cereal is a great way to start the day.

¼ cup amaranth flour
¼ cup millet flour
¼ cup brown rice grits or yellow corn grits (polenta)
¼ cup tahini, almond butter, or peanut butter
Pinch sea salt
3 cups water, plus more as needed
Pure maple syrup (optional)
Gluten-free plain or vanilla nondairy milk (optional)

Put the amaranth flour, millet flour, grits, tahini, and salt in a large, heavy saucepan. Gradually whisk in the water until smooth. Bring to a gentle simmer over medium-high heat. Decrease the heat to low and cook uncovered, stirring almost constantly with the whisk, until thick and creamy, 20 to 25 minutes. Constant stirring is necessary to prevent lumps, burning, or sticking. Add more water if the mixture becomes too thick. Serve hot, sweetened with maple syrup to taste and topped with milk as desired.

Per serving: 223 calories, 7 g protein, 13 g fat (2 g sat), 21 g carbs, 29 mg sodium, 31 mg calcium, 3 g fiber

amaranth breakfast cereal

Hot amaranth cereal makes a terrific addition to any breakfast repertoire. Its naturally nutty flavor pairs beautifully with fresh berries.

1 cup amaranth

2½ cups water

Pinch ground cinnamon

Pinch ground nutmeg

Pinch sea salt

½ cup gluten-free plain or vanilla nondairy milk, plus more as needed

1 cup fresh blueberries or sliced strawberries

½ cup chopped toasted walnuts

Pure maple syrup

Put the amaranth in a medium saucepan. Add the water, cinnamon, nutmeg, and salt and bring to a boil over high heat. Decrease the heat to medium-low, partially cover, and cook, stirring occasionally, until all the water is absorbed, 25 to 30 minutes. Gradually stir in the milk, adding more if necessary to achieve the desired consistency, and heat through. Serve hot, topped with the blueberries and walnuts. Drizzle with maple syrup if desired.

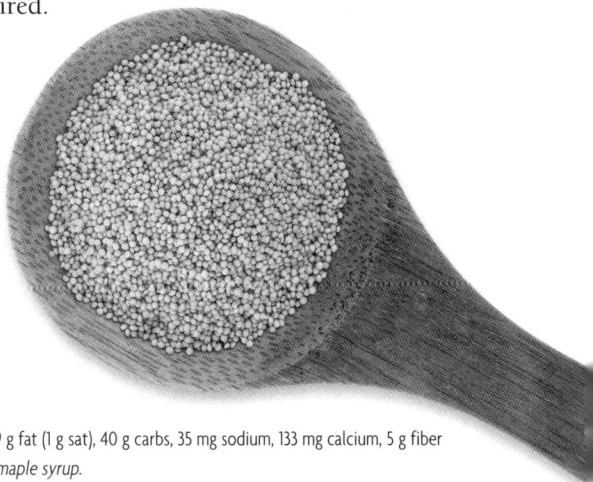

Per serving: 260 calories, 8 g protein, 9 g fat (1 g sat), 40 g carbs, 35 mg sodium, 133 mg calcium, 5 g fiber
Note: Analysis does not include pure maple syrup.

quick quinoa hot cereal

This creamy hot cereal is made with quick-cooking quinoa flakes, so it can be on the table in under five minutes. Because quinoa is a rich source of protein, this dish makes a hearty, nutritious breakfast.

2 cups gluten-free plain or vanilla nondairy milk

¾ cup quinoa flakes

Pinch sea salt

Sliced banana

Chopped toasted walnuts, peanut butter, or gluten-free
    vegan butter

Pure maple syrup

Put the milk in a medium saucepan and bring to a boil over medium-high heat. Add the quinoa flakes and salt and stir to combine. Remove from the heat, cover, and let sit undisturbed for 3 minutes to let the quinoa absorb the liquid and thicken. Stir well. Serve topped with banana, walnuts, and maple syrup as desired.

Per serving: 227 calories, 6 g protein, 5 g fat (0 g sat), 40 g carbs, 262 mg sodium, 450 mg calcium, 4 g fiber
Note: Analysis does not include banana, walnuts, or pure maple syrup.

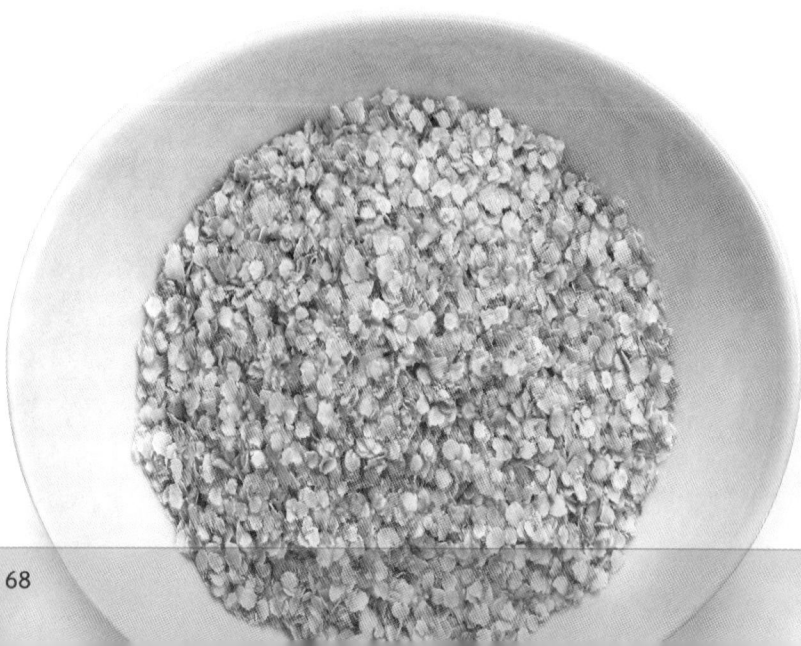

rice and raisin pudding

MAKES 4 SERVINGS

This wholesome, not-too-sweet pudding is made with arborio rice, a short-grain Italian rice with a high starch content. It's traditionally used for making risotto because its starch gives that classic Italian dish its characteristic creaminess. For the same reason, arborio rice is ideal for making lusciously creamy rice pudding. Don't rinse arborio rice before using it, as doing so will wash away the essential starch. Serve this pudding warm or chilled for breakfast or dessert. It also makes a great between-meal snack.

3½ cups gluten-free vanilla nondairy milk
½ cup arborio rice
¼ cup raisins
¼ cup pure maple syrup
Pinch sea salt
Ground cinnamon (optional)

Put the milk, rice, raisins, maple syrup, and salt in a medium saucepan and bring to a boil over medium-high heat. Decrease the heat to low and gently simmer uncovered, stirring frequently, until the rice is tender and the liquid is thickened and creamy, about 45 minutes. Garnish with a sprinkle of cinnamon if desired.

TIP: The pudding will continue to thicken as it cools. For an even creamier pudding, increase the milk to 4 cups and extend the cooking time to 1 hour.

VARIATION: For an even richer, creamier pudding, use lite or regular coconut milk in place of some or all of the milk and add 1 teaspoon of gluten-free vanilla extract.

Per serving: 265 calories, 3 g protein, 2 g fat (0 g sat), 59 g carbs, 138 mg sodium, 404 mg calcium, 2 g fiber

breakfast grits

This Southern breakfast staple is a tasty alternative to cooked cereals that contain gluten. Serve it savory style, with just a touch of vegan butter and a sprinkle of pepper, or on the sweet side, topped with toasted seeds, maple syrup, and nondairy milk.

GRITS

4½ cups water

1 cup yellow corn grits (polenta) or brown rice grits

½ teaspoon sea salt

OPTIONAL TOPPINGS

Gluten-free vegan butter, extra-virgin olive oil, or coconut butter

Freshly ground black pepper

Toasted pumpkin or sunflower seeds

Pure maple syrup, brown sugar, or fruit preserves

Gluten-free plain nondairy milk or lite coconut milk

Put the water, grits, and salt in a heavy saucepan and bring to a boil over medium-high heat, stirring frequently. Decrease the heat to low, cover, and cook, stirring occasionally, until thick, 15 to 20 minutes. Remove from the heat and let stand, covered, to thicken a little more, 3 to 5 minutes. The longer the grits stand, the thicker they will get. Serve hot with the toppings of your choice.

SCRAMBLED GRITS: Chill Breakfast Grits (without toppings) in a sealed container in the refrigerator for 8 to 12 hours or longer. The grits will become very firm. Mince or shred your favorite vegetables and cook them in a large skillet (preferably nonstick) in olive oil or coconut oil until tender. Add the cold grits, breaking them into chunks with the side of a spoon. Season with salt and pepper and your favorite fresh or dried herbs and/or gluten-free hot sauce, chili powder, or curry powder to taste. For a heartier meal, add cooked or canned beans, drained. Cook and stir over medium-high heat until the grits are hot and lightly browned.

Per serving: 140 calories, 2 g protein, 1 g fat (0 g sat), 31 g carbs, 225 mg sodium, 0 mg calcium, 3 g fiber
Note: Analysis does not include optional toppings.

salad bar

chilled noodles in a spicy sauce

Saucy chilled noodles are irresistibly enticing. And because they're served cold, they make a lovely and convenient addition to a buffet or party meal as an appetizer or main dish.

NOODLE SALAD

½ cup tahini or almond butter

2 tablespoons balsamic vinegar

2 tablespoons toasted hot sesame oil, chili oil, or extra-virgin olive oil

1 tablespoon freshly squeezed lemon juice or lime juice

2 teaspoons peeled and grated fresh ginger, or ½ teaspoon ground ginger

1 teaspoon pure maple syrup (optional)

½ teaspoon minced or pressed garlic

Water, as needed

Gluten-free hot sauce

Sea salt

12 ounces gluten-free spaghetti

VEGGIE ADDITIONS (CHOOSE THREE)

Carrots, grated

English cucumber, thinly sliced

Jalapeño chile, seeded and minced

Red, yellow, orange, or green bell peppers, cut into matchsticks

Red or green cabbage, grated or very thinly sliced

Red radishes, thinly sliced

Water chestnuts or jicama, sliced or diced

OPTIONAL TOPPINGS

Green onions, thinly sliced

Fresh cilantro or flat-leaf parsley, chopped

Raw or toasted sesame seeds, pumpkin seeds, sunflower seeds, or slivered almonds

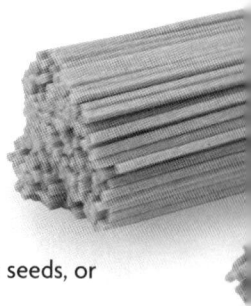

Put the tahini, vinegar, oil, lemon juice, ginger, optional maple syrup, and garlic in a large bowl. Stir vigorously until smooth and well combined. Gradually whisk in enough water to make a pourable sauce, about 1 cup, beating vigorously until completely smooth. Season with hot sauce and salt to taste.

Cook the spaghetti in boiling water according to the package directions. Drain in a colander. Rinse well under cold water, then drain again. Add to the bowl with the sauce along with the veggie additions of your choice and toss until the noodles are coated and the ingredients are evenly distributed. Taste and add more hot sauce or salt if desired. Cover tightly and refrigerate until well chilled before serving, at least 2 hours. The noodles will absorb any excess sauce as they chill. Garnish with the optional toppings as desired.

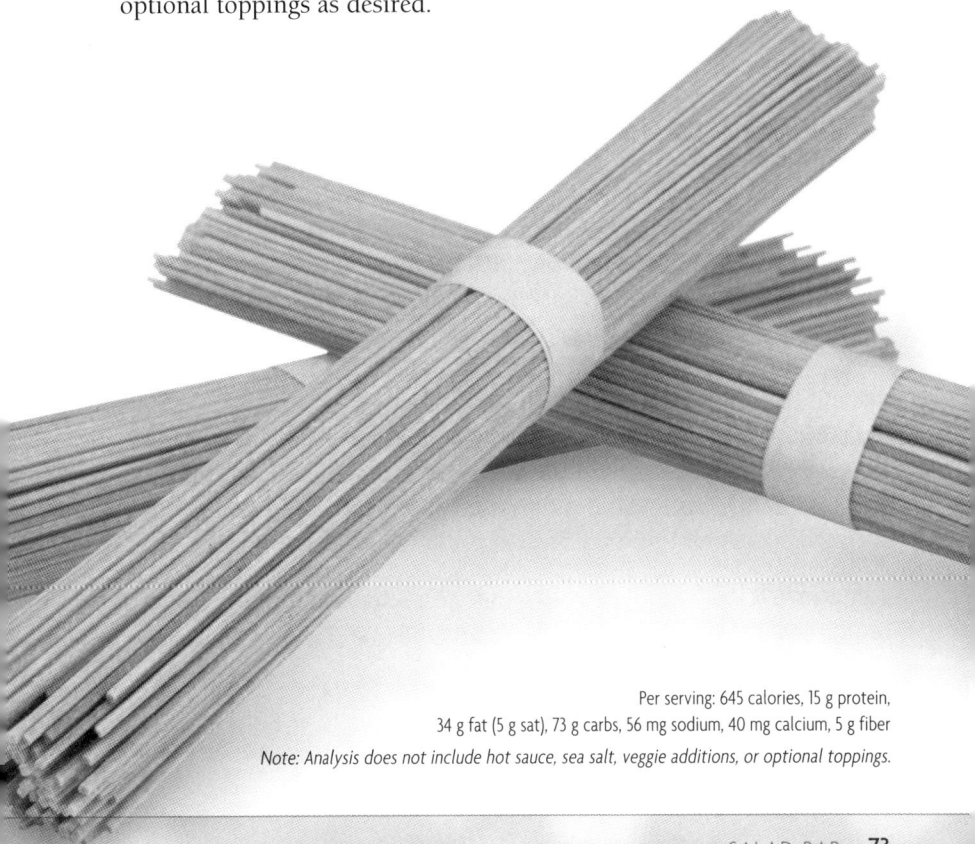

Per serving: 645 calories, 15 g protein,
34 g fat (5 g sat), 73 g carbs, 56 mg sodium, 40 mg calcium, 5 g fiber
Note: Analysis does not include hot sauce, sea salt, veggie additions, or optional toppings.

warm peanut noodles with snow peas

Although this salad is best served warm or at room temperature, chilled leftovers make an awesome packed lunch or picnic meal. Peanut butter and toasted sesame oil impart an enchanting flavor and aroma.

1 pound gluten-free linguine, fettuccine, or spaghetti
3 tablespoons toasted sesame oil or hot sesame oil
½ pound snow peas, trimmed
½ cup smooth or chunky peanut butter
3 tablespoons freshly squeezed lime juice
1 teaspoon minced or pressed garlic
Reduced-sodium tamari
Cayenne or gluten-free hot sauce
1 English cucumber, diced or cut into thin half-moons
2 green onions, thinly sliced

Cook the linguine in boiling water according to the package directions. Drain in a colander. Rinse well under cold water, then drain again. Transfer to a large bowl, add the sesame oil, and toss until evenly coated. (The oil will help keep the noodles from sticking together).

While the linguine is cooking, fill a medium saucepan halfway with water and bring to a boil over high heat. Add the snow peas and cook for 1 minute. Drain in a colander, let cool, and cut crosswise into thirds.

Put the peanut butter, lime juice, and garlic in a small bowl. Stir to combine. Whisk in just enough water, about ½ cup, to make a thick but pourable sauce. Season with tamari and cayenne to taste. Pour over the cooked linguine. Add the snow peas, cucumber, and green onions and toss gently until the noodles are coated and the vegetables are evenly distributed. Serve warm or at room temperature.

VARIATION: Omit the snow peas. Add ½ cup halved and thinly sliced or diced red radishes along with the cucumber and green onions.

Per serving: 476 calories, 11 g protein, 17 g fat (3 g sat), 71 g carbs, 89 mg sodium, 62 mg calcium, 5 g fiber
Note: Analysis does not include reduced-sodium tamari, cayenne, or hot sauce.

sorghum salad with chickpeas and roasted grape tomatoes

Packed with protein and flavor, this light salad features roasted grape tomatoes and a mild lemony dressing. It's hearty enough to be a complete meal.

1 pint grape or cherry tomatoes

3 tablespoons extra-virgin olive oil

¼ teaspoon plus a pinch sea salt

3 cups cooked sorghum (see table, page 26)

1½ cups no-salt-added cooked or canned chickpeas, drained

¼ cup sliced oil-cured or kalamata olives

2 tablespoons freshly squeezed lemon juice

¼ teaspoon crushed red pepper flakes

1 clove garlic, minced or pressed

Freshly ground black pepper

3 cups baby arugula, lightly packed

Preheat the oven to 400 degrees F. Line a rimmed baking sheet or small roasting pan with parchment paper or a silicone baking mat.

Put the tomatoes in a medium bowl. Add 1 tablespoon of the oil and a pinch of salt. Toss gently. Transfer to the lined baking sheet and bake until soft and starting to burst, 15 to 20 minutes.

Put the sorghum, chickpeas, and olives in a large bowl and stir gently to combine.

Put the remaining 2 tablespoons of oil and the lemon juice, red pepper flakes, garlic, and remaining ¼ teaspoon of salt in a small bowl and whisk to combine. Pour over the sorghum mixture. Add the tomatoes and their juices and toss gently until evenly combined. Season with pepper to taste and toss again. Arrange the arugula on a platter and top with the salad mixture.

Per serving: 451 calories, 13 g protein, 15 g fat (2 g sat), 69 g carbs, 254 mg sodium, 67 mg calcium, 15 g fiber

roasted brussels sprouts and rice salad

Even if you're not a big fan of Brussels sprouts, you will love this salad. Roasting brings out the natural sweetness of Brussels sprouts and makes them irresistible. The bright, lively seasonings in this dish complement them perfectly.

1 pound Brussels sprouts, trimmed and quartered, if large, or halved, if small

1 tablespoon extra-virgin olive oil, melted coconut oil, or other neutral oil

½ teaspoon sea salt, plus more as needed

½ teaspoon freshly ground black pepper

2¼ cups water

1 cup brown rice or brown and wild rice blend

2 tablespoons freshly squeezed lemon or lime juice or red wine vinegar, plus more as needed

2 tablespoons toasted or hot sesame oil

1 tablespoon balsamic vinegar

1 teaspoon peeled and grated fresh ginger

Garlic powder

Sea salt

2 roasted or fresh red bell peppers, diced or sliced into matchsticks

½ cup raw or toasted sunflower or pumpkin seeds, pignolia nuts, or slivered almonds (optional)

Preheat the oven to 400 degrees F.

Put the Brussels sprouts, olive oil, salt, and pepper in a large roasting pan (preferably nonstick) and toss until the Brussels sprouts are evenly coated with the oil and salt. Spread into a single layer. Roast in the oven for 40 to 45 minutes, stirring every 15 minutes and spreading into a single layer again, until the sprouts are crisp, brown, and tender. Transfer to a large bowl.

While the Brussels sprouts are roasting, put the water and rice in a large saucepan and bring to a boil over high heat. Cover, decrease the heat to low, and cook until the water is absorbed and the rice is tender, 45 to 50 minutes. Remove from the heat and let rest, covered, for 10 minutes. Transfer to a large bowl and add the Brussels sprouts, lemon juice, sesame oil, vinegar, and ginger and stir to combine. Season with garlic powder and salt to taste. Add more lemon juice to taste if desired. Serve warm, garnished with the red bell peppers and sunflower seeds if desired.

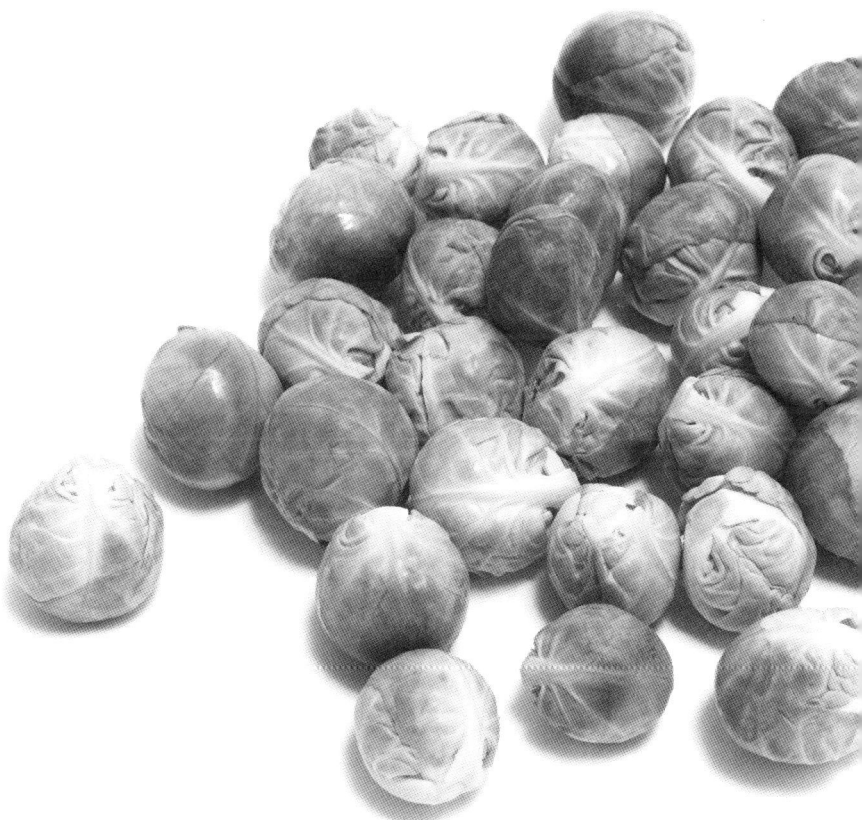

Per serving: 330 calories, 7 g protein, 13 g fat (2 g sat), 47 g carbs, 256 mg sodium, 50 mg calcium, 7 g fiber

roasted cauliflower and radishes

This unusual combination is a game changer. Roasting brings out the best in cauliflower and takes radishes, which are typically served raw, to an entirely different plane.

 4 cups cauliflower florets

 15 red radishes, trimmed and halved lengthwise

 2 tablespoons extra-virgin olive oil, melted coconut oil, or other neutral oil

 ½ teaspoon sea salt

 ½ teaspoon freshly ground black pepper

 1 teaspoon grated lemon zest

 1 teaspoon freshly squeezed lemon juice, plus more as needed

 ½ cup chopped fresh cilantro or flat-leaf parsley, lightly packed

Preheat the oven to 400 degrees F.

Put the cauliflower, radishes, olive oil, salt, and pepper in a large roasting pan (preferably nonstick) and toss until the vegetables are evenly coated with the oil and salt. Spread into a single layer. Roast in the oven for 35 to 40 minutes, stirring every 15 minutes and spreading into a single layer again, until the vegetables are crisp, brown, and tender. Transfer to a medium bowl. Add the lemon zest and lemon juice and toss until evenly distributed. Taste and add more lemon juice if desired. Serve warm, garnished with the cilantro.

Per serving: 88 calories, 3 g protein, 7 g fat (1 g sat), 6 g carbs, 264 mg sodium, 31 mg calcium, 3 g fiber

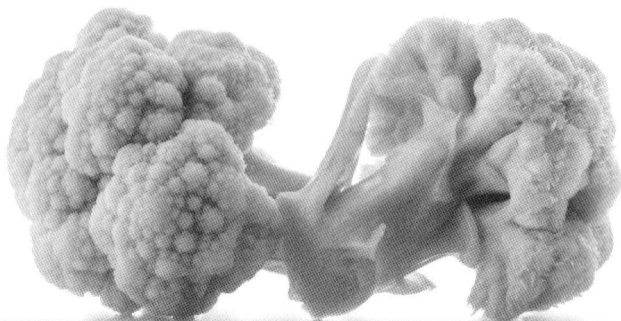

curried rice and fruit salad with apricot dressing

Apricot preserves make a light and flavorful foundation for the salad dressing in this recipe, while the unique combination of fruits and seasonings creates an exotic and delightful taste sensation.

4 cups water

2 cups white basmati rice

2 tablespoons organic canola oil, safflower oil, or other neutral oil

1 tablespoon gluten-free curry powder

1 tablespoon peeled and grated fresh ginger

1 teaspoon sea salt

½ teaspoon minced or pressed garlic

2 crisp apples, diced (peeling optional)

1½ cups crushed pineapple packed in juice, well drained

1 ripe banana, sliced

½ cup chopped fresh cilantro or flat-leaf parsley, lightly packed

⅓ cup unsweetened shredded dried coconut

1 tablespoon dried mint

½ cup fruit-sweetened apricot preserves

2 tablespoons freshly squeezed lemon juice

Cayenne

Put the water, rice, 1 tablespoon of the oil, and the curry powder, ginger, salt, and garlic in a large saucepan and bring to a boil over high heat. Decrease the heat to low, cover, and cook until the rice is tender and the water is absorbed, 15 to 20 minutes. Remove from the heat and let stand, covered, for 10 minutes. Fluff with a fork and let cool.

Transfer the cooled rice to a large bowl. Add the apples, pineapple, banana, cilantro, coconut, and mint and stir to combine. Put the preserves, lemon juice, and remaining tablespoon of oil in a small bowl and stir or whisk until well combined. Pour over the rice mixture. Season with cayenne to taste. Serve immediately.

Per serving: 415 calories, 5 g protein, 9 g fat (3 g sat), 71 g carbs, 311 mg sodium, 20 mg calcium, 3 g fiber
Note: Analysis does not include cayenne.

mediterranean dilled vegetable and rice salad

MAKES 6 SERVINGS

Kalamata olives and dill weed add a lot of flavor to this salad, so a light dressing suits it quite well. To effortlessly turn this dish into a delicious main course, serve it on a fluffy bed of baby arugula or spring mix.

3 cups water
1½ cups long-grain white or basmati rice
3 tomatoes, diced
1 medium zucchini, diced
1 red bell pepper, diced
1 cup frozen peas, cooked and drained
⅔ cup sliced kalamata olives
¼ cup diced red onion
3 tablespoons freshly squeezed lemon juice
2 tablespoons extra-virgin olive oil
1 tablespoon dried dill weed
Sea salt
Freshly ground black pepper

Put the water in a medium saucepan and bring to a boil over medium-high heat. Stir in the rice, cover, decrease the heat to low, and cook until the rice is tender and the water is absorbed, 15 to 20 minutes. Remove from the heat and let stand, covered, for 10 minutes. Fluff with a fork and let cool.

Transfer the cooled rice to a large bowl. Add the tomatoes, zucchini, bell pepper, peas, olives, onion, lemon juice, oil, and dill weed and toss gently until well combined. Season with salt and pepper to taste. Serve immediately.

Per serving: 308 calories, 4 g protein, 10 g fat (1 g sat), 50 g carbs, 512 mg sodium, 12 mg calcium, 3 g fiber
Note: Analysis does not include sea salt or freshly ground black pepper.

tri-color quinoa-corn salad

Quinoa turns this tasty salad into a satisfying meal. The multitude of colors from the vegetables make it especially appetizing.

1½ cups water

1 cup quinoa, rinsed well and drained

2 cups fresh or frozen corn kernels, cooked, or canned corn, drained

1 red bell pepper, finely diced

½ cup thinly sliced green onions

¼ cup extra-virgin olive oil

3 tablespoons freshly squeezed lemon juice

2 teaspoons gluten-free Dijon mustard

Sea salt

Freshly ground black pepper

Put the water in a medium saucepan and bring to a boil over high heat. Stir in the quinoa, cover, and decrease the heat to low. Cook until all the water is absorbed and the grain is tender, about 25 minutes. Remove from the heat and let stand, covered, for 5 minutes. Fluff with a fork, then transfer to a large bowl. Stir in the corn, bell pepper, and green onions. Put the oil, lemon juice, and mustard in a small bowl and whisk until well combined. Pour over the quinoa mixture and toss gently. Season with salt and pepper to taste. Serve warm, chilled, or at room temperature.

Per serving: 383 calories, 8 g protein, 17 g fat (2 g sat), 48 g carbs, 51 mg sodium, 29 mg calcium, 4 g fiber
Note: Analysis does not include sea salt or freshly ground black pepper.

quinoa tabbouleh

Classic Middle Eastern tabbouleh is traditionally made with bulgur wheat, but quinoa makes a spectacular alternative. Because quinoa is a nutritional powerhouse loaded with protein, you can easily serve this salad in larger portions as a scrumptious main course. For an even heartier salad, try the variation.

1½ cups water
1 cup quinoa, rinsed well and drained
2 tablespoons freshly squeezed lemon juice
1 clove garlic, minced or pressed
¼ cup extra-virgin olive oil
1 large English cucumber, diced
1 pint cherry tomatoes, halved
⅔ cup chopped flat-leaf parsley, firmly packed
2 green onions, thinly sliced
¼ cup chopped fresh mint, firmly packed, or 1 tablespoon
  dried mint
Sea salt
Freshly ground black pepper

Put the water in a medium saucepan and bring to a boil over high heat. Stir in the quinoa, cover, and decrease the heat to low. Cook until all the water is absorbed and the grain is tender, about 25 minutes. Remove from the heat and let stand, covered, for 5 minutes. Fluff with a fork, then transfer to a large bowl and let cool to room temperature, fluffing it occasionally with a fork to speed the process.

To make the dressing, put the lemon juice and garlic in a small bowl. Gradually whisk in the oil until the mixture is emulsified.

When the quinoa is cool, add the cucumber, tomatoes, parsley, green onions, and mint and toss gently to combine. Whisk the dressing again and pour over the salad. Toss gently until evenly mixed. Season with salt and pepper to taste.

VARIATION: To make this salad a substantial main dish, add 1½ cups of cooked or canned chickpeas, drained, along with 1 cup of halved and thinly sliced red radishes and/or 1 cup of shredded carrots.

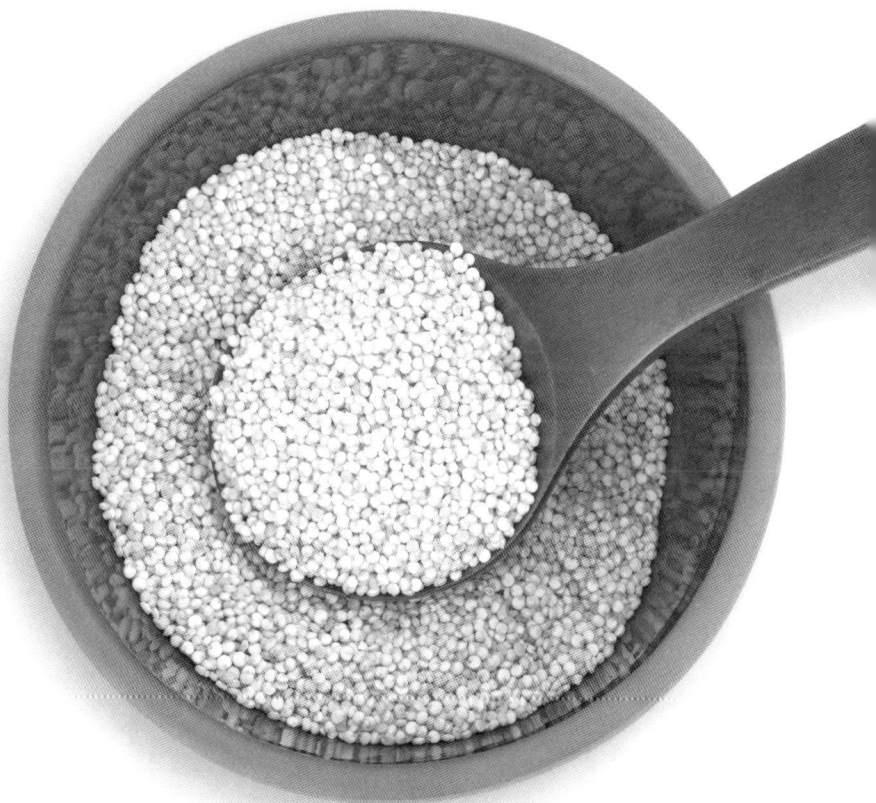

Per serving: 161 calories, 5 g protein, 7 g fat (1 g sat), 23 g carbs, 9 mg sodium, 34 mg calcium, 3 g fiber
Note: Analysis does not include sea salt or freshly ground black pepper.

baby kale salad
with pine nuts and blueberries

Baby kale is not only a nutritional powerhouse but it's also sweet and tender, making it a fantastic salad green. When combined with blueberries and pine nuts, kale is elevated beyond its well-established superfood status. This salad is loaded with taste as well as plentiful antioxidants, calcium, and vitamins A, C, and K.

2 tablespoons freshly squeezed lemon juice

2 teaspoons Dijon mustard

3 tablespoons extra-virgin olive oil

Sea salt

Freshly ground black pepper

4 cups baby kale, lightly packed

1 cup blueberries

¼ cup pine nuts, lightly toasted

To make the dressing, put the lemon juice and mustard in a small bowl and gradually whisk in the oil, beating vigorously until emulsified. Season with salt and pepper to taste.

To make the salad, put the kale, blueberries, and pine nuts in a large bowl. Whisk the dressing again, pour over the salad, and toss until evenly distributed. Serve immediately.

Per serving: 188 calories, 3 g protein, 16 g fat (2 g sat), 12 g carbs, 79 mg sodium, 51 mg calcium, 2 g fiber
Note: Analysis does not include sea salt or freshly ground black pepper.

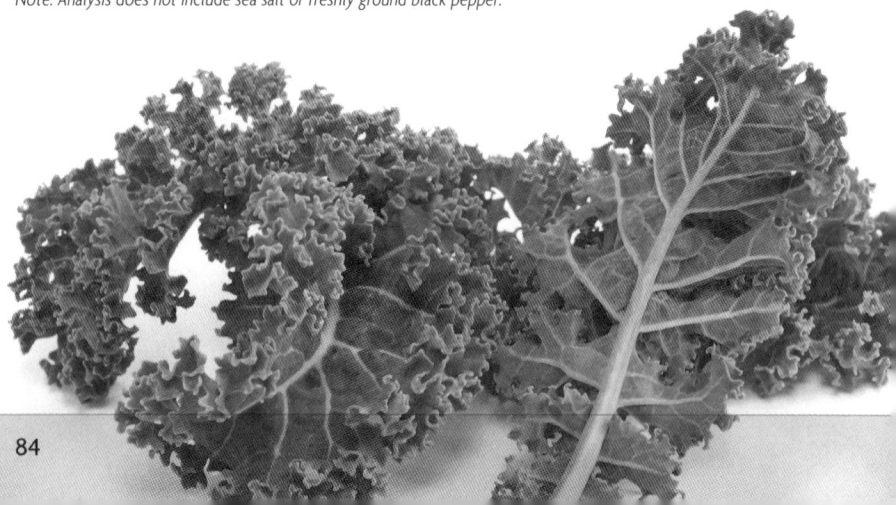

citrus fruit and grain salad

Tart and juicy, this scrumptious salad uses fresh fruit and pantry staples to create the centerpiece of a meal.

4 cups cooked brown rice, basmati rice, wild rice, quinoa, or a combination (see table, page 26), cooled to room temperature

2 navel oranges, cut into bite-sized pieces

½ cup minced flat-leaf parsley, lightly packed

⅓ cup sliced dates or raisins

¼ cup extra-virgin olive oil

3 tablespoons freshly squeezed lemon juice

1 tablespoon red wine vinegar, white wine vinegar, or balsamic vinegar

2 teaspoons gluten-free Dijon mustard

Sea salt

Freshly ground black pepper

Put the rice, oranges, parsley, and dates in a large bowl and stir gently to combine. Put the oil, lemon juice, vinegar, and mustard in a small bowl and whisk until well combined. Pour over the rice mixture and toss until evenly distributed. Season with salt and pepper to taste. Serve chilled or at room temperature.

Per serving: 274 calories, 4 g protein, 11 g fat (2 g sat), 43 g carbs, 47 mg sodium, 37 mg calcium, 4 g fiber

Note: Analysis does not include sea salt or freshly ground black pepper.

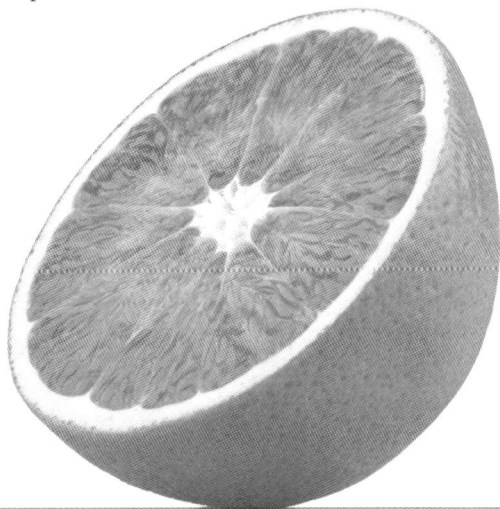

ruby wild rice salad

This salad fills the bill for holiday gatherings and other special occasions, although it's great for everyday meals as well. It's made with dried cranberries, which look like glistening rubies. Radishes and seeds add a pleasing crunch.

3 cups water or gluten-free vegetable broth
1 cup wild rice
1¼ cups diced daikon radish or other radishes
1 cup dried cranberries
1 orange, yellow, or red bell pepper, diced
1 cup lightly toasted sunflower or pumpkin seeds
½ cup sliced green onions
⅓ cup orange juice
2 tablespoons balsamic vinegar
2 tablespoons extra-virgin olive oil
1 teaspoon gluten-free Dijon mustard
Sea salt
Freshly ground pepper

Put the water in a medium saucepan and bring to a boil. Stir in the wild rice, cover, and decrease the heat to medium-low. Cook until the rice kernels puff open and are butterflied, 50 to 60 minutes. Drain off any excess liquid. Transfer to a large bowl and let cool to room temperature, fluffing it occasionally with a fork to speed the process.

Add the radish, cranberries, bell pepper, sunflower seeds, and green onions to the wild rice and toss to combine. Put the orange juice, vinegar, olive oil, and mustard in a small measuring cup or bowl and whisk until well combined. Pour over the wild rice mixture and toss gently until evenly distributed. Season with salt and pepper to taste. Serve chilled or at room temperature.

Per serving: 559 calories, 15 g protein, 28 g fat (4 g sat), 69 g carbs, 187 mg sodium, 68 mg calcium, 8 g fiber
Note: Analysis does not include sea salt or freshly ground black pepper.

sorghum and white bean salad

Sorghum pearls are about the same size as Israeli couscous, but they're gluten-free and provide a lot more nutritional value. Sorghum has a chewy texture similar to wheat berries, but its flavor is milder.

DRESSING

2 tablespoons freshly squeezed lemon or lime juice

1 teaspoon gluten-free Dijon mustard

1 clove garlic, minced or pressed

¼ cup extra-virgin olive oil

SALAD

3 cups cooked sorghum (see table, page 26), cooled until warm

1½ cups no-salt-added cooked or canned white beans, drained

2 green onions, thinly sliced

Sea salt

Freshly ground black pepper

4 cups baby kale or baby spinach leaves, lightly packed

To make the dressing, combine the lemon juice, mustard, and garlic in a small bowl and whisk to combine. Gradually whisk in the oil, beating vigorously until emulsified.

To make the salad, put the sorghum in a large bowl. Add the beans and green onions and toss to combine. Add the dressing and toss until evenly distributed. Season with salt and pepper to taste. Arrange the kale on a platter and top with the sorghum salad.

Per serving: 486 calories, 14 g protein, 16 g fat (2 g sat), 79 g carbs, 49 mg sodium, 120 mg calcium, 16 g fiber
Note: Analysis does not include sea salt or freshly ground black pepper.

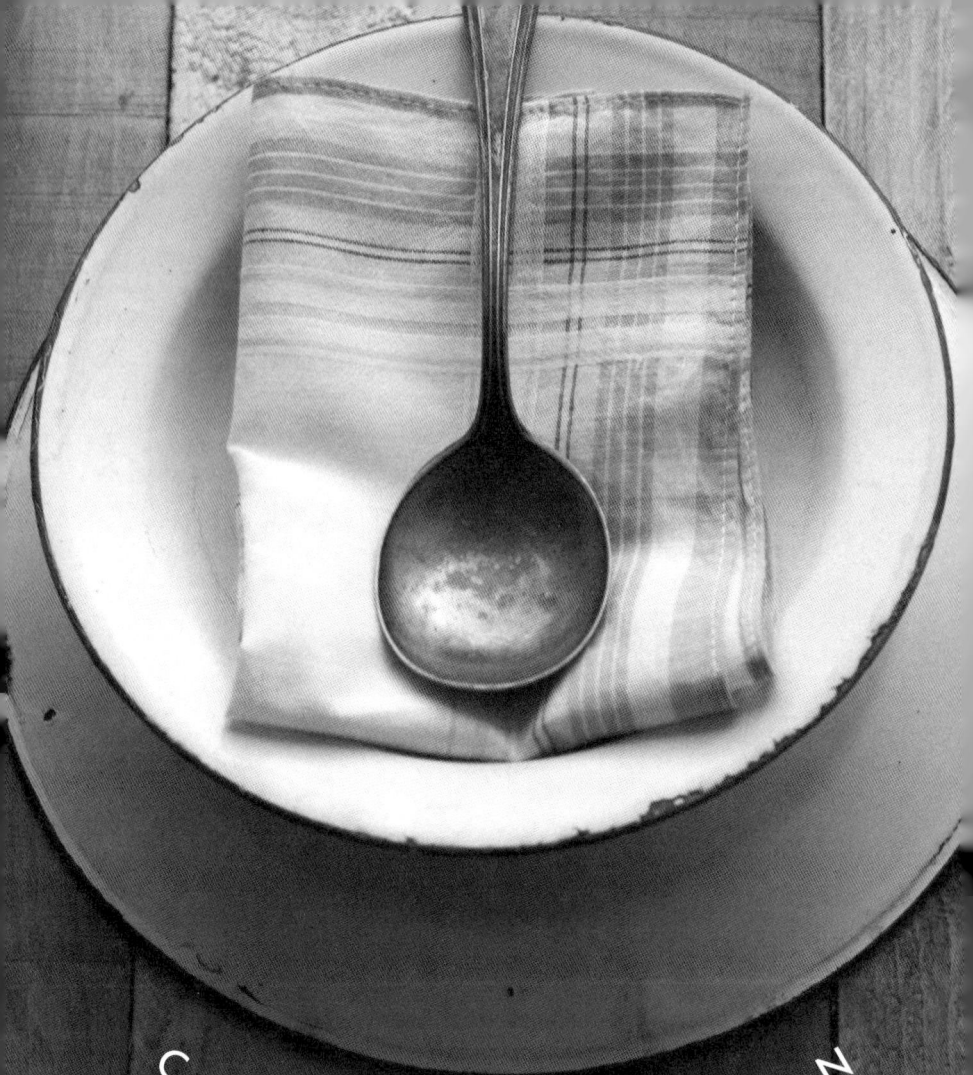

10

soup kettle

lentil and rice soup

Simple ingredients make for a hearty lentil soup that's out of this world. It's high in protein and healthful complex carbohydrates, a combination that will give you staying power. The slow-cooked onions are the secret to this soup's compelling flavor.

8 cups water or gluten-free vegetable broth, plus more as needed
1 cup dried lentils, rinsed and drained
1 cup diced or chopped carrots
½ cup brown rice
¼ cup extra-virgin olive oil
1 large onion, chopped
Sea salt
Freshly ground pepper

Put the water, lentils, carrots, and rice in a large soup pot and bring to a boil over high heat. Decrease the heat to medium-low, cover, and simmer, stirring occasionally, until the lentils are very tender and the soup is thick, 1½ to 2 hours. If the soup becomes too thick, add a little extra water.

While the soup is cooking, put the oil in a large skillet over medium-high heat. When hot, add the onion and cook, stirring frequently, until very tender and brown, 30 to 60 minutes. Decrease the heat as necessary so the onion doesn't burn. Add the onion and any remaining oil in the skillet to the soup. Season with salt and pepper to taste. Partially cover and simmer, stirringly occasionally, for 10 to 15 minutes longer to allow the flavors to blend.

Per 1 cup: 149 calories, 5 g protein, 7 g fat (1 g sat), 22 g carbs, 14 mg sodium, 9 mg calcium, 6 g fiber
Note: Analysis does not include sea salt or freshly ground black pepper.

cream of cauliflower and lima bean soup

MAKES 8 CUPS

This creamy soup has a portion of whole lima beans added for extra texture. Even though it's thick and rich tasting, the soup contains no flour or added starches. Use only frozen Fordhook lima beans, which are large, sweet, and meaty.

1 package (1 pound) frozen Fordhook lima beans
1 tablespoon extra-virgin olive oil
1½ cups chopped onions
2 teaspoons whole caraway seeds, or 1½ teaspoons ground caraway seeds
1 teaspoon minced or pressed garlic
1 medium cauliflower, cut into small florets
5 cups water or gluten-free vegetable broth
Sea salt
Freshly ground black pepper
Chopped fresh cilantro or flat-leaf parsley, for garnish

Cook the lima beans until tender according to the package directions. Drain.

Put the oil in a large soup pot over medium-high heat. When hot, add the onions, caraway seeds, and garlic and cook, stirring frequently, until the onions are soft, 10 to 15 minutes. Add the cauliflower and water and bring to a boil over high heat. Decrease the heat to medium-low, cover, and simmer until the cauliflower is very tender, 10 to 12 minutes.

Process the soup in batches in a blender along with half the lima beans. Return the blended soup to the pot and stir in the remaining whole lima beans. Season with salt and pepper to taste. Warm over medium-low heat until the beans are heated through and the soup is steaming hot. Garnish with cilantro just before serving.

Per 1 cup: 117 calories, 5 g protein, 3 g fat (1 g sat), 16 g carbs, 86 mg sodium, 38 mg calcium, 6 g fiber
Note: Analysis does not include sea salt or freshly ground black pepper.

white bean and cabbage soup

This delectable recipe uses common, inexpensive ingredients to create a delicious soup that's both satisfying and nutritious.

2 tablespoons extra-virgin olive oil

1 large onion, chopped

1 teaspoon minced or pressed garlic

8 cups water or gluten-free vegetable broth

3 cups no-salt-added cooked or canned white beans, drained

1 small head green cabbage, finely chopped

8 ounces butternut squash or other winter squash, peeled and cubed

1 teaspoon dried thyme

Sea salt

Freshly ground black pepper

Put the oil in a large soup pot and heat over medium-high heat. When hot, add the onion and cook, stirring frequently, until it begins to brown, about 15 minutes. Decrease the heat as necessary so the onion doesn't burn. Add the garlic and cook, stirring frequently, for 1 minute. Add the water, beans, cabbage, squash, and thyme. Increase the heat to high and bring to a boil. Decrease the heat to medium-low, cover, and cook, stirring occasionally, until the squash is very tender and the flavors have blended, about 1 hour. Season with salt and pepper to taste.

Per 1 cup: 131 calories, 6 g protein, 3 g fat (0.3 g sat), 25 g carbs, 20 mg sodium, 86 mg calcium, 5 g fiber
Note: Analysis does not include sea salt or freshly ground black pepper.

quick broccoli bisque

This quick and satisfying soup is creamy but not heavy. It's a super-rich source of nutrients but is virtually fat-free, as its creaminess is derived from blended beans rather than dairy products or flour.

8 cups coarsely chopped broccoli florets

7 cups water or gluten-free vegetable broth

2 cups coarsely chopped celery

1 large onion, coarsely chopped

2 teaspoons dried basil

1 teaspoon minced or pressed garlic

3 cups no-salt-added cooked or canned white beans, drained

Sea salt

Freshly ground black pepper

Put the broccoli, water, celery, onion, basil, and garlic in a large soup pot and bring to a boil over high heat. Decrease the heat to medium, cover, and simmer until the vegetables are tender, about 15 minutes. Process with the beans in batches in a blender until smooth. Return the blended mixture to the soup pot, season with salt and pepper to taste, and simmer over medium-high heat, stirring occasionally, until hot.

Per 1 cup: 100 calories, 7 g protein, 1 g fat (0 g sat), 17 g carbs, 66 mg sodium, 79 mg calcium, 6 g fiber
Note: Analysis does not include sea salt or freshly ground black pepper.

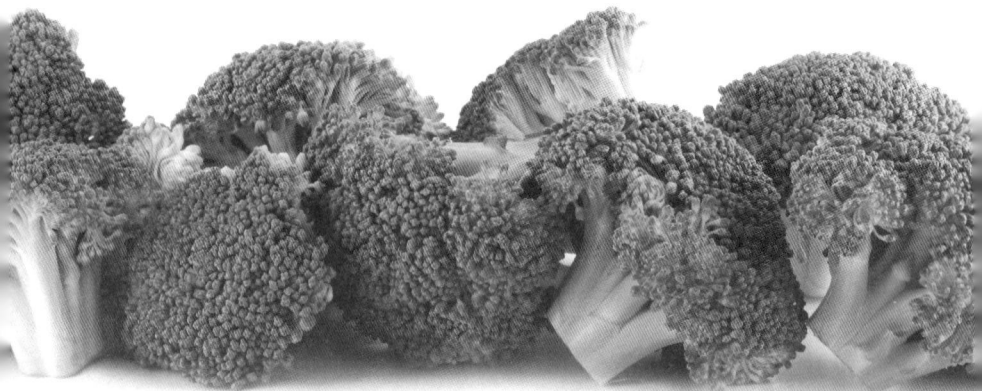

creamy carrot bisque with exotic spices

Although there are no dairy products or flour in this exotically flavored soup, the texture is incredibly creamy. In addition to beta-carotene, which gives the soup its vivid color, it's rich in a wide range of minerals, including chromium, copper, magnesium, manganese, molybdenum, phosphorus, and potassium.

2 tablespoons extra-virgin olive oil
1 large onion, coarsely chopped
1 pound carrots, peeled and sliced
1 large potato, peeled and coarsely chopped
½ teaspoon ground cardamom
½ teaspoon ground cinnamon
¼ teaspoon ground ginger
¼ teaspoon ground nutmeg
7 cups water or gluten-free vegetable broth
Sea salt
Cayenne

Put the oil in a large soup pot over medium-high heat. When hot, add the onion and cook, stirring frequently, for 5 minutes. Stir in the carrots and potato and stir until coated with the oil. Decrease the heat to medium and stir in the cardamom, cinnamon, ginger, and nutmeg. Cook, stirring frequently, for 10 minutes. Add the water, increase the heat to medium-high, and bring to a boil. Decrease the heat to medium-low, cover, and simmer until the vegetables are very tender, about 30 minutes. Process in batches in a blender until smooth. Return the blended mixture to the soup pot, season with salt and cayenne to taste, and simmer over medium-high heat, stirring occasionally, until hot.

Per 1 cup: 110 calories, 2 g protein, 4 g fat (1 g sat), 18 g carbs, 49 mg sodium, 37 mg calcium, 3 g fiber
Note: Analysis does not include sea salt or freshly ground black pepper.

purée of parsnips and leeks

The delicate, sweet taste of parsnips is enlivened by the oniony flavor of leeks and the peppery bite of ginger in this light and creamy soup.

1 tablespoon extra-virgin olive oil
1 cup sliced leeks (see tip)
1 tablespoon peeled and grated fresh ginger, or 1 teaspoon ground ginger
4 cups water or gluten-free vegetable broth
1½ pounds parsnips, peeled and coarsely chopped
1 cup unsweetened plain nondairy milk, heated, or hot water
Sea salt
Paprika, for garnish

Put the oil in a large soup pot over medium-high heat. When hot, add the leeks and cook, stirring frequently, for 5 minutes. Add the ginger and cook, stirring constantly, for 1 minute. Add the water and parsnips and bring to a boil. Decrease the heat to medium, cover, and simmer, stirring occasionally, until the parsnips are very tender, 20 to 25 minutes.

Process the soup in batches in a blender until smooth. Return the blended soup to the soup pot and stir in the hot milk. Warm the soup, stirring almost constantly, until it is just heated through, about 5 minutes. Season with salt to taste. Garnish each serving with a light dusting of paprika.

TIP: Rinse leeks thoroughly to remove the sandy grit and dirt that tends to hide in the leaves. To do this, lay each leek horizontally on a cutting board, with the root in one hand and your knife in the other. Make a horizontal cut lengthwise from the bulb to the green end. Separate the leaves gently so the inner sections are exposed and rinse well under running water. Alternatively, slice the leek crosswise, separate the slices into rings, put in a colander, and rinse well under running water. Use only the white bulb and tender green section (the lower part) of the leek, as the dark-green upper portion will be tough.

Per 1 cup: 121 calories, 2 g protein, 3 g fat (0.4 g sat), 23 g carbs, 37 mg sodium, 86 mg calcium, 6 g fiber
Note: Analysis does not include sea salt or paprika.

millet chili

This hearty chili is a quick solution for busy weekday dinners or cold-weather get-togethers.

1 tablespoon extra-virgin olive oil
1 large onion, diced
1 green bell pepper, diced
4 cloves garlic, minced or pressed
1 jalapeño chile, seeded and finely chopped
1 teaspoon gluten-free chili powder
1 teaspoon ground cumin
1 teaspoon sea salt
1 teaspoon freshly ground black pepper
3 cups no-salt-added cooked or canned red beans, drained
2 cups fresh or frozen corn kernels
4 cups no-salt-added gluten-free vegetable broth or water
1 cup millet
1 can (15 ounces) no-salt-added diced tomatoes, with juice
1 can (6 ounces) no-salt-added tomato paste

Put the oil in a large saucepan and heat over medium heat. When hot, add the onion, bell pepper, garlic, and chile and cook, stirring frequently, until the onion is soft and translucent, about 10 minutes. Stir in the chili powder, cumin, salt, and pepper. Add the beans and corn and stir to combine. Add the broth, increase the heat to medium-high, and bring to a boil. Stir in the millet. Decrease the heat to medium-low, cover, and cook, stirring occasionally, for 30 minutes. Add the tomatoes with their juice and the tomato paste and stir until the paste is well incorporated. Simmer uncovered, stirring occasionally, until the millet is tender and the flavors have blended, about 15 minutes.

Per 1 cup: 263 calories, 9 g protein, 3 g fat (1 g sat), 47 g carbs, 293 mg sodium, 53 mg calcium, 9 g fiber

gravy boat

11

savory chickpea gravy

This handy sauce is a delicious way to enhance even the simplest meals. Folks who swear they don't like beans will love it. Since it's made with toasted chickpea flour, they'll never know they're eating beans.

> 3 tablespoons extra-virgin olive oil
> 1 cup chickpea flour
> 1 teaspoon rubbed sage
> ½ teaspoon dried rosemary, crumbled
> ½ teaspoon dried thyme, crumbled
> ¼ teaspoon freshly ground black pepper
> 3½ cups hot water, plus more as needed
> 1½ tablespoons umeboshi vinegar
> 1 tablespoon balsamic vinegar
> Sea salt

Put the oil in a large saucepan over medium heat. When hot, add the flour, sage, rosemary, thyme, and pepper, stirring constantly to form a smooth, thick paste. Cook, stirring almost constantly, until the flour is lightly toasted and no longer tastes raw, 8 to 10 minutes. Remove from the heat. Gradually whisk in the hot water, beating vigorously to avoid lumps. Whisk in the umeboshi vinegar and balsamic vinegar. Warm over medium heat, whisking occasionally, until hot and bubbly. Season with salt to taste and whisk in additional water, if needed, to achieve the desired consistency.

Per ¼ cup: 53 calories, 2 g protein, 3 g fat (0.4 g sat), 12 g carbs, 5 mg sodium, 0 mg calcium, 1 g fiber
Note: Analysis does not include sea salt.

great gravy

This versatile gravy is terrific on all savory foods, from beans to biscuits to mashed potatoes to meatless meats.

¼ cup arrowroot or cornstarch
1 tablespoon balsamic vinegar
1 tablespoon umeboshi vinegar
3¼ cups water or gluten-free vegetable broth
1 teaspoon garlic powder
¼ cup tahini
Sea salt

Put the arrowroot, balsamic vinegar, and umeboshi vinegar in a medium saucepan. Mix well to make a smooth paste. Gradually whisk in the water and garlic powder. Cook over medium-high heat, whisking constantly, until the gravy thickens and comes to a boil, about 5 minutes. Remove from the heat and whisk in the tahini, beating vigorously until smooth. Season with salt to taste. Serve at once.

TIP: This makes a very thick gravy. If you prefer a thinner sauce, gradually whisk in additional water, 1 teaspoon at a time, until you achieve the desired consistency.

Per ¼ cup: 54 calories, 2 g protein, 4 g fat (1 g sat), 9 g carbs, 1 mg sodium, 8 mg calcium, 1 g fiber
Note: Analysis does not include sea salt.

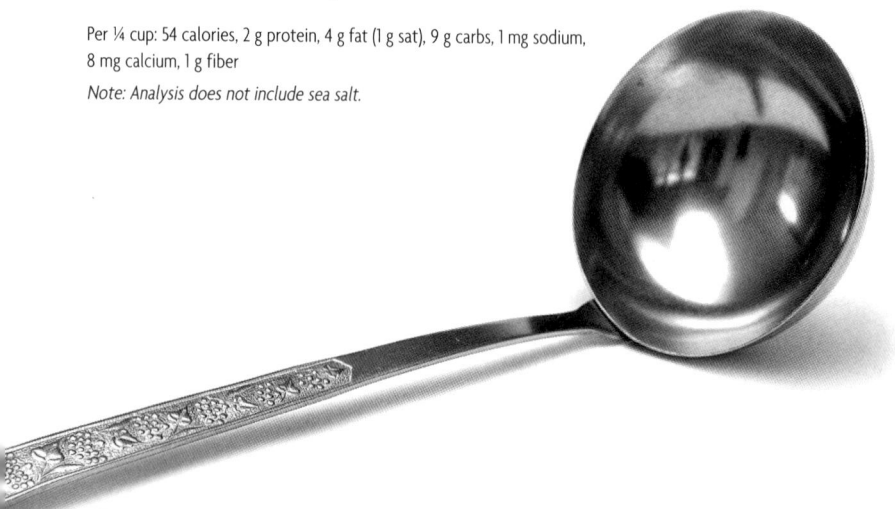

everyday mushroom gravy

MAKES 4 CUPS

Most people save gravy for holiday meals and other special occasions. But gravy is such a delicious condiment, why not enjoy it other times as well? This version is so tasty you'll want to pour it over tempeh, tofu, baked or mashed potatoes, roasted or steamed veggies, and, of course, gluten-free biscuits.

2 tablespoons extra-virgin olive oil
1 cup minced onion
¼ teaspoon rubbed sage
¼ teaspoon dried thyme
1 teaspoon minced or pressed garlic
8 ounces mushrooms, stemmed and finely chopped
½ teaspoon sea salt
2 tablespoons cornstarch
4 cups no-salt-added gluten-free vegetable broth or water
Tamari
Freshly ground black pepper

Put the oil in a medium saucepan over medium-high heat. When hot, add the onion, sage, and thyme and cook, stirring frequently, until the onion is soft and translucent, about 10 minutes. Add the garlic and cook, stirring almost constantly, for 1 minute. Add the mushrooms and salt and stir to evenly distribute. Decrease the heat to medium-low, cover, and cook, stirring occasionally, until the mushrooms are tender and have released their juices.

Put the cornstarch in a small bowl and gradually whisk in 1 cup of the broth, beating vigorously until smooth. Pour the remaining 3 cups of broth into the mushroom mixture. Increase the heat to medium-high and bring to a boil. Decrease the heat to medium-low and gradually drizzle in the cornstarch mixture, stirring constantly. Cook, stirring frequently, until glossy and thickened, about 10 minutes. Season with tamari and pepper to taste.

Per ¼ cup: 28 calories, 0 g protein, 2 g fat (0.3 g sat), 3 g carbs, 57 mg sodium, 5 mg calcium, 1 g fiber
Note: Analysis does not include tamari or freshly ground black pepper.

miso white sauce

This effortless sauce is quite luscious and can be used in place of white sauce in most conventional recipes. It's fabulous spooned over tempeh or tofu and makes a terrific topping for rice-and-veggie bowls.

⅓ cup tahini
¼ cup gluten-free chickpea miso
2 tablespoons freshly squeezed lemon juice
¾ cup hot water, as needed

Put the tahini, miso, and lemon juice in a small bowl and stir well to make a thick paste. Gradually stir or whisk in the water, using just enough water to achieve the desired consistency and beating vigorously after each addition until smooth and creamy. To warm the sauce further, transfer to a small saucepan and briefly heat over medium-low heat, stirring frequently, for about 1 minute. Do not boil.

Per ¼ cup: 164 calories, 6 g protein, 12 g fat (2 g sat), 8 g carbs, 408 mg sodium, 22 mg calcium, 2 g fiber

12

main event

black bean tostadas

Enjoy this south-of-the-border specialty with plenty of your favorite toppings and create a party in your mouth.

TOSTADAS

2 cups no-salt-added cooked or canned black beans, drained

1 tablespoon freshly squeezed lime juice

2 teaspoons gluten-free chili powder

1 teaspoon garlic powder

½ teaspoon ground cumin

½ teaspoon dried oregano

Sea salt

Gluten-free hot sauce

8 corn tortillas or Gluten-Free Chapatis (page 58)

1 tablespoon extra-virgin olive oil

½ cup finely chopped onion

TOPPING OPTIONS (SELECT TWO OR MORE)

Avocado, cut into chunks

Black olives, sliced

Carrots, shredded

Cilantro, chopped

Green onions, sliced

Lettuce, shredded

Red onion, chopped

Salsa

Tomatoes, chopped

Coarsely chop the beans by hand or by pulsing them briefly in a food processor. Put the beans, lime juice, chili powder, garlic powder, cumin, and oregano in a medium bowl and stir to combine. Season with salt and hot sauce to taste.

Warm the tortillas one by one in a large skillet over medium heat, then stack them on a clean towel and fold the towel over them to keep them warm. Put the oil in the skillet and increase the heat to medium-high. When hot, add the onion and cook, stirring frequently, until very tender, 10 to 15 minutes. Add the bean mixture and cook, stirring frequently, until warmed through and starting to brown, about 5 minutes. Spoon an equal portion of the bean mixture onto each of the tortillas. Add your favorite toppings or put bowls of several different toppings on the table. To eat, gently fold the tortillas and pick up the tostadas with your hands.

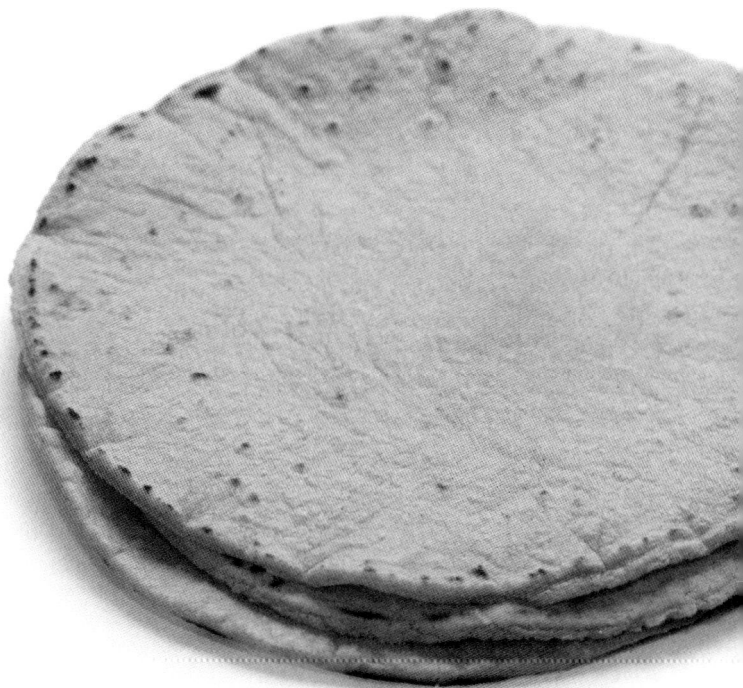

Per serving: 252 calories, 9 g protein, 6 g fat (1 g sat), 41 g carbs, 103 mg sodium, 9 mg calcium, 10 g fiber
Note: Analysis does not include sea salt, hot sauce, or topping options.

brown rice patties

This recipe calls for short-grain brown rice because the almost-round kernels tend to be sticky and cling together, especially when the rice is freshly cooked. Leftover cooked patties can be stored in a sealed container in the freezer. Use food wrap or parchment paper to separate them before packing them in the container.

> 2 cups cooked short-grain brown rice (see table, page 26)
> 1 cup shredded carrots
> ½ cup finely chopped onion
> ½ cup chopped fresh cilantro or flat-leaf parsley, lightly packed
> 1 teaspoon sea salt
> ½ teaspoon minced or pressed garlic
> ¼ teaspoon freshly ground pepper
> ½ cup GF All-Purpose Flour Mix (page 36) or other gluten-free all-purpose flour

Put the rice, carrots, onion, parsley, salt, garlic, and pepper in a large bowl. Add the flour mix and stir until evenly distributed. If the mixture doesn't hold together, add up to ¼ cup of water, 1 tablespoon at a time, until it does, taking care to not add any more water than is necessary. Form into 12 patties, firmly pressing the patties with your hands, using about ¼ cup per patty. Coat a large, heavy skillet (preferably nonstick) with oil and heat over medium heat. When hot, cook the patties in batches, depending on the size of the skillet, until brown on the bottom, 5 to 7 minutes. Turn and brown the other side, about 5 minutes. Add more oil to the skillet between each batch.

Per patty: 65 calories, 1 g protein, 0 g fat (0 g sat), 14 g carbs, 151 mg sodium, 7 mg calcium, 1 g fiber

igor's special

This quick pasta dish is not only delicious but it also can be on the table in a flash. It's a convenient staple to keep in your weekly rotation, and the quantities can easily be doubled if you need to increase the number of servings. I prefer corn spaghetti in this dish, but rice spaghetti or any other gluten-free pasta will work just as well.

6 ounces gluten-free spaghetti or other gluten-free pasta
2 cups fresh or frozen bite-sized broccoli florets, thawed
1 large, ripe tomato, chopped
¼ cup sliced green onions or chopped red onion
¼ cup coarsely chopped walnuts or whole pumpkin or sunflower seeds
1 tablespoon balsamic vinegar
1 tablespoon extra-virgin olive oil
1 tablespoon freshly squeezed lemon juice
¼ teaspoon minced or pressed garlic
¼ teaspoon gluten-free curry powder
Cayenne
Umeboshi vinegar or sea salt
Freshly ground black pepper

Fill a large soup pot halfway with water and bring to a boil. Add the spaghetti, decrease the heat to medium-high, and cook, stirring frequently, until just barely tender. Do not drain. Remove the pot from the heat and add the broccoli florets. Cover and let rest until the spaghetti and broccoli are tender, 5 to 8 minutes.

While the pasta and broccoli are resting, put the tomato, green onions, walnuts, balsamic vinegar, oil, lemon juice, garlic, and curry powder in a large bowl.

Drain the spaghetti and broccoli in a colander. Rinse well under cold water, then drain again. Transfer to the bowl with the tomato and toss gently but thoroughly. Season with cayenne, umeboshi vinegar, and pepper to taste.

Per serving: 472 calories, 11 g protein, 14 g fat (1 g sat), 77 g carbs, 32 mg sodium, 51 mg calcium, 5 g fiber
Note: Analysis does not include cayenne, umeboshi vinegar, or freshly ground black pepper.

moroccan millet

This pilaf makes a terrific one-dish meal on its own, or serve it with a fresh green salad on the side.

2 tablespoons extra-virgin olive oil
1 large red bell pepper, cut into strips
1 large green bell pepper, cut into strips
1 large onion, cut into half-moons
2 tablespoons minced or pressed garlic
2 teaspoons paprika
½ teaspoon sea salt
1 teaspoon ground cumin
½ teaspoon ground cinnamon
¼ teaspoon cayenne
¼ teaspoon ground ginger
¼ teaspoon ground turmeric
1½ cups millet
3 cups water or gluten-free vegetable broth
1¾ cups no-salt-added cooked or canned chickpeas, drained
¼ cup raisins or chopped dates
¼ cup pine nuts, pumpkin seeds, or sunflower seeds (optional)
Sea salt
Freshly ground black pepper

Preheat the oven to 450 degrees F.

Put 1 tablespoon of the oil in a large roasting pan. Add the red bell pepper, green bell pepper, onion, garlic, paprika, and salt. Stir until the vegetables are evenly coated with the oil. Roast the vegetables for 20 minutes, stirring two or three times partway through the cooking cycle. Let cool, then chop the vegetables coarsely.

While the vegetables are roasting, heat the remaining tablespoon of oil in a large saucepan. Add the cumin, cinnamon, cayenne, ginger, and turmeric. Cook over medium-high heat, stirring constantly, until the spices are uniform in color and well combined, about 30 seconds. Add the millet, stir quickly to coat with the spices, and cook, stirring constantly, for 1 minute. Immediately pour in the water and bring to a boil. Decrease the heat to low, cover, and cook until all the liquid is absorbed and the millet is tender, about 30 minutes.

Transfer the millet to a large bowl and fluff with a fork. Add the roasted vegetables, chickpeas, raisins, and optional pine nuts. Toss gently to combine. Season with salt and pepper to taste.

Per serving: 415 calories, 12 g protein, 12 g fat (1 g sat), 67 g carbs, 87 mg sodium, 47 mg calcium, 11 g fiber
Note: Analysis does not include additional sea salt or freshly ground black pepper.

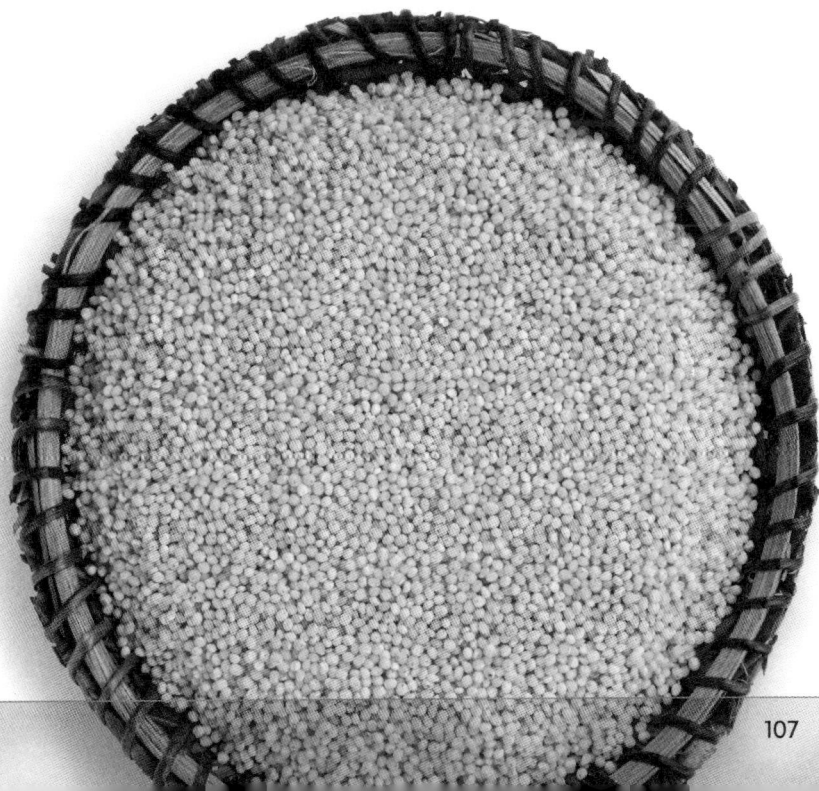

quinoa primavera

Because quinoa cooks so quickly, this beautiful composition can be pulled together in record time, yet it never fails to impress. Frozen peas are recommended because they're so handy, but you can certainly use lightly steamed garden-fresh peas if you're fortunate enough to have those on hand.

1½ cups water
1 cup quinoa, rinsed well and drained
2 cups frozen green peas, thawed and drained
2 tablespoons extra-virgin olive oil
2 carrots, peeled and thinly sliced on the diagonal
2 zucchini, thinly sliced on the diagonal
1 red bell pepper, diced or cut into thin strips
1 green bell pepper, diced or cut into thin strips
2 large leeks, thinly sliced (see tip, page 94)
1 teaspoon minced or pressed garlic
2 teaspoons dried dill weed
Sea salt
Freshly ground black pepper

Put the water in a large saucepan and bring to a boil over high heat. Stir in the quinoa, cover, and decrease the heat to low. Cook until the quinoa is tender and the water is absorbed, about 25 minutes. Remove from the heat and scatter the peas on top of the quinoa; do not stir. Cover and let rest for 8 minutes.

While the quinoa rests, put the oil in a large skillet over medium-high heat. When hot, add the carrots, zucchini, red bell pepper, green bell pepper, leeks, and garlic. Cook, stirring frequently, until the carrots are tender-crisp, about 10 minutes. Add the quinoa, peas, and dill weed and toss gently until well combined. Heat over medium heat, tossing constantly, until the peas are heated through, about 2 minutes. Season with salt and pepper to taste.

Per serving: 358 calories, 13 g protein, 10 g fat (1 g sat), 57 g carbs, 124 mg sodium, 80 mg calcium, 11 g fiber
Note: Analysis does not include sea salt or freshly ground black pepper.

chickpea flour pizza

This unusual dish is a cross between a soft, tender pizza crust and a high-protein flatbread. It's simple to prepare and tastes amazing. If you have chickpea flour on hand, it's a snap to make. Serve it with a side of sliced tomatoes, a salad, or a vegetable dish for a complete meal. Although it's delish on its own, it can be turned into a full-fledged pizza simply by layering on your favorite pizza toppings during the last part of cooking.

½ cup chickpea flour
¼ teaspoon dried basil, crumbled between your fingers
¼ teaspoon dried oregano, crumbled between your fingers
¼ teaspoon garlic powder
¼ teaspoon sea salt
Generous pinch cayenne or freshly ground black pepper
Pinch ground turmeric
½ cup water
1 teaspoon extra-virgin olive oil

Put the chickpea flour, basil, oregano, garlic powder, salt, cayenne, and turmeric in a medium bowl. Gradually whisk in the water, beating vigorously after each addition until completely smooth. Generously oil a heavy, 10-inch skillet (preferably nonstick) or mist it well with cooking spray and heat over medium-high heat. When hot, stir the batter and pour it into the pan, scraping all of it out with a silicone spatula. Drizzle the olive oil over the top. Cook until the top is set and the bottom is nicely browned, 5 to 7 minutes. Adjust the heat as necessary to prevent overbrowning. Carefully turn the pizza over and cook the other side until well browned, about 5 minutes. Slide onto a round plate and slice into 8 wedges. Serve immediately.

Per serving: 300 calories, 11 g protein, 17 g fat (2 g sat), 27 g carbs, 470 mg sodium, 16 mg calcium, 5 g fiber

spinach and herb frittata

The secret to the eggy flavor of this crustless quiche is the black salt, also known as *kala namak*. This salt originates from India, and despite its name, it's pink, not black. Black salt contains sulfur, which gives it a distinctive egg-like aroma and taste. Look for it at Indian grocery stores or specialty shops or order online (see tip).

1½ cups chickpea flour
½ teaspoon freshly ground black pepper
½ teaspoon ground turmeric
¼ teaspoon gluten-free baking powder
¼ teaspoon sea salt
¼ teaspoon gluten-free black salt or additional sea salt
¼ teaspoon cayenne
2 cups water
2 tablespoons extra-virgin olive oil
2 cups chopped spinach or stemmed Swiss chard, lightly packed
1 cup chopped onion
½ cup chopped flat-leaf parsley, lightly packed
½ cup chopped fresh cilantro or additional parsley, lightly packed
2 tablespoons chopped fresh dill, or 1 teaspoon dried dill weed

Preheat the oven to 375 degrees F. Generously oil a 10-inch ovenproof skillet (preferably nonstick or cast iron).

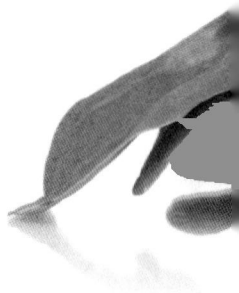

Put the chickpea flour, pepper, turmeric, baking powder, sea salt, black salt, and cayenne in a large bowl and whisk to combine. Gradually whisk in the water, beating vigorously until lump-free and completely smooth. Whisk in 1 tablespoon of the oil until well blended. Add the spinach, onion, parsley, cilantro, and dill and stir until well combined. Pour into the oiled skillet, scraping out the bowl with a silicone spatula. Bake for 20 to 25 minutes, until the top is firm, lightly browned, and starting to crack. Drizzle evenly with the remaining tablespoon of oil and bake for 5 minutes longer. Let cool for 10 to 15 minutes before slicing.

TIP: Look for gluten-free black salt online from Saltworks (saltworks. us), Spice Jungle (spicejungle.com), and Uncle Harry's Natural Products (uncleharrys.com).

Per serving: 147 calories, 6 g protein, 6 g fat (1 g sat), 17 g carbs, 204 mg sodium, 38 mg calcium, 4 g fiber

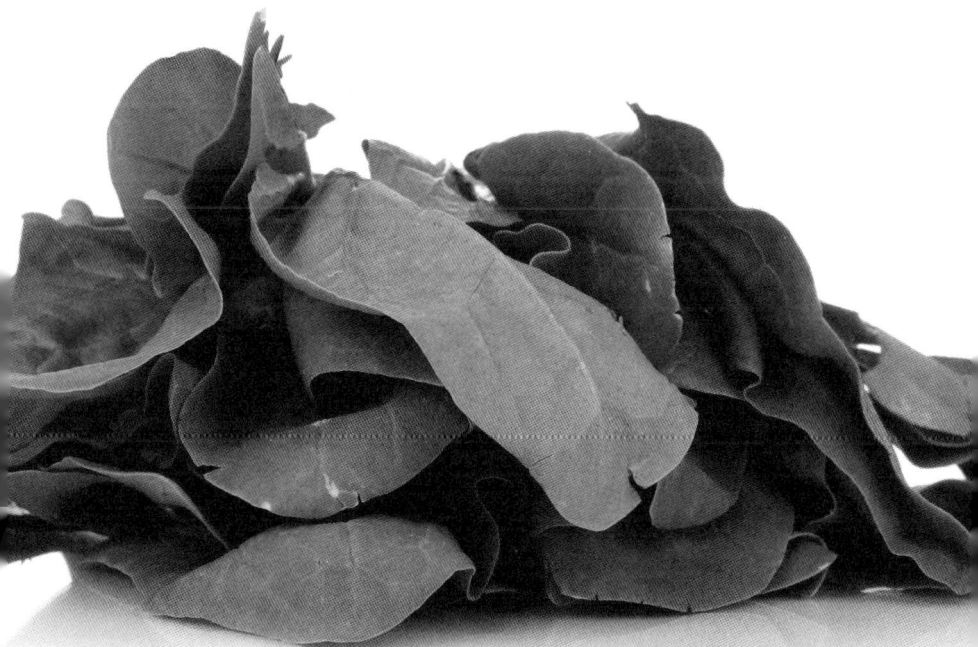

spinach and chickpea curry

Rich and spicy, this exquisite stew tastes like it has been cooking all day, yet it can be ready and on the table in mere minutes. Serve it alongside basmati or jasmine rice and a cooling cucumber salad.

1½ tablespoons coconut oil

1 cup chopped onion

1 teaspoon minced or pressed garlic

2 teaspoons gluten-free chili powder

2 teaspoons ground coriander

2 teaspoons ground cumin

1 teaspoon ground cinnamon

1 teaspoon ground turmeric

½ teaspoon freshly ground black pepper

⅔ cup water

½ cup no-salt-added tomato paste

2 teaspoons unbleached cane sugar

6 cups baby spinach, lightly packed

3 cups no-salt-added cooked or canned chickpeas, drained

Sea salt

Put the oil in a large skillet or soup pot and heat over medium-high heat. When hot, add the onion and cook, stirring frequently, until very tender and brown, about 15 minutes. Add the garlic, and cook, stirring frequently, for 1 minute. Decrease the heat to medium and stir in the chili powder, coriander, cumin, cinnamon, turmeric, and pepper. Cook, stirring constantly, for 30 seconds.

Add the water, tomato paste, and sugar and stir until well combined. Stir in the spinach and chickpeas. Cook, stirring almost constantly, until the spinach is wilted and the beans are heated through, about 5 minutes. Season with salt to taste.

Per serving: 294 calories, 14 g protein, 9 g fat (5 g sat), 44 g carbs, 201 mg sodium, 174 mg calcium, 13 g fiber
Note: Analysis does not include sea salt.

veggie rice roll

This is such a fun, easy-to-transport, gluten-free "sandwich." Serve it with your favorite gluten-free dipping sauce.

1 **rice paper sheet** (about 8½ inches in diameter)

⅓ **cup cooked rice** (any kind)

1 tablespoon **gluten-free barbecue sauce, plum sauce, peanut sauce, or other gluten-free sauce,** plus more for serving

3 slices **avocado**

2 tablespoons **grated carrot**

2 tablespoons **raw or lightly toasted pumpkin or sunflower seeds** (optional)

2 tablespoons **diced gluten-free baked tofu or cooked or canned beans, drained** (optional)

¼ cup **alfalfa sprouts or chopped romaine lettuce**

Fresh **basil leaves, mint leaves, or cilantro** (optional)

Fill a large bowl with warm water. Dip the rice paper sheet into the water for 5 seconds, then put it on a cutting board. Pat it with a dry cloth to absorb excess water. Put the rice in the center of the sheet, then cover it with the sauce, avocado, carrot, optional pumpkin seeds, optional tofu, sprouts, and optional basil. Fold the right and left margins of the rice paper toward the center. Then fold up the bottom margin. Fold the top margin down, using a bit of pressure to seal the roll. Serve with additional sauce for dipping as desired.

Per serving: 244 calories, 3 g protein, 5 g fat (2 g sat), 46 g carbs, 290 mg sodium, 14 mg calcium, 4 g fiber

creamy quiche

This simple quiche is easily adapted to a number of variations. It contains no eggs, cream, cow's milk, or cheese, yet it's very creamy and rich tasting. Serve it with thick slices of fresh tomato on the side and hot steamed greens for a hearty and memorable meal.

1 recipe (one crust) **Pat-in-the-Pan Pie Crust** (page 40)

3 cups no-salt-added cooked or canned white beans, drained

¾ cup full-fat coconut milk

½ cup **GF All-Purpose Flour Mix** (page 36) or other gluten-free all-purpose flour

½ cup water

1 tablespoon gluten-free chickpea miso

¼ teaspoon sea salt

¼ teaspoon gluten-free black salt or additional sea salt

¼ teaspoon ground nutmeg

¼ teaspoon ground turmeric

1 tablespoon extra-virgin olive oil, coconut oil, or organic canola oil

1 large onion, finely chopped

Preheat the oven to 400 degrees F.

Prebake the pie crust for 14 minutes. Let cool. Keep the oven on but decrease the temperature to 350 degrees F.

Put the beans, coconut milk, flour mix, water, miso, salt, black salt, nutmeg, and turmeric in a blender or food processor and process several minutes until the mixture is completely smooth. Stop frequently to stir the mixture and scrape down the container with a silicone spatula. Set aside.

Put the oil in a medium skillet over medium-high heat. When hot, add the onion and cook, stirring frequently, until tender and golden, about 12 minutes. Stir into the blended mixture and pour into the prebaked pie crust. Bake on the center rack of the oven for about 1 hour, or until the top is firm, browned, and slightly puffed. Let rest for 15 to 20 minutes before slicing.

TIP: The quiche will continue to firm up as it cools, and leftovers will get very firm when chilled in the refrigerator. Because of this, it makes an excellent packed lunch.

BROCCOLI QUICHE: Steam 2 cups of bite-sized broccoli florets until tender. Stir them into the blended mixture just before pouring into the prebaked pie crust. Bake as directed.

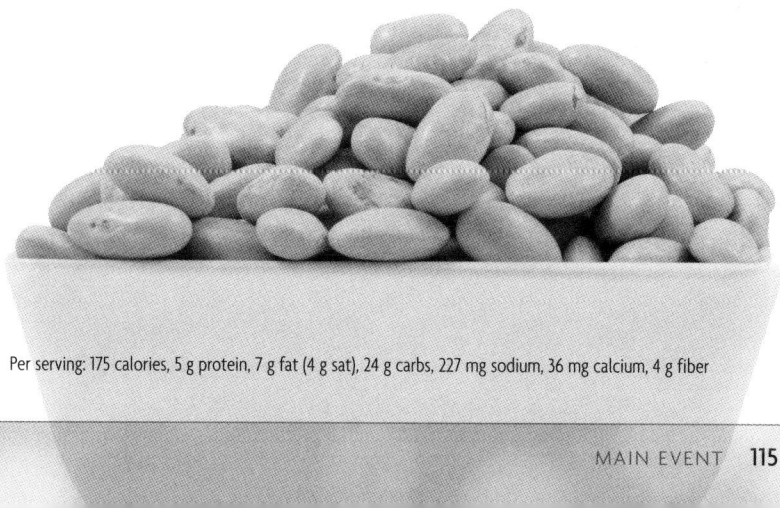

GREEN ONION OR CHIVE QUICHE: Omit the onion and oil. Stir ½ cup of thinly sliced green onions or chives into the blended mixture just before pouring into the prebaked pie crust. Bake as directed. This variation may be used in combination with any of the other variations.

HERB QUICHE: Omit the nutmeg. Stir 2 tablespoons of fresh herbs or 2 teaspoons of dried herbs into the blended mixture. Good choices include basil, dill weed, marjoram, oregano, rosemary, sage, or thyme, or a combination of two or more. If desired, cook ½ to 1 teaspoon of minced or pressed garlic along with the onion.

MUSHROOM QUICHE: Add 2 cups of sliced mushrooms to the onion once the onion is soft, and continue cooking until the mushrooms are tender and almost all of the liquid has evaporated. Stir into the blended mixture just before pouring into the prebaked pie crust. Bake as directed.

Per serving: 175 calories, 5 g protein, 7 g fat (4 g sat), 24 g carbs, 227 mg sodium, 36 mg calcium, 4 g fiber

pad thai mashup

This unique take on pad thai incorporates a delicious combination of flavors from Italy, Japan, and Thailand. The result is superb! For an ideal side dish to accompany it, try a colorful medley of steamed vegetables, such as broccoli florets, diagonally sliced carrots, red bell pepper strips, and sliced water chestnuts.

12 ounces rice fettuccine

¼ cup no-salt-added tomato paste

¼ cup brown rice vinegar

¼ cup water

2 tablespoons pure maple syrup

2 tablespoons toasted sesame oil

1 tablespoon gluten-free chickpea miso

2 teaspoons gluten-free hot chili sauce, or 1 teaspoon crushed red pepper flakes

½ teaspoon minced or pressed garlic

¼ cup fresh cilantro leaves, packed

¼ cup thinly sliced green onions

¼ cup coarsely chopped gluten-free unsalted roasted peanuts

Cook the fettuccine in boiling water according to the package directions. Drain well and transfer to a large bowl.

While the fettuccine is cooking, put the tomato paste, vinegar, water, maple syrup, oil, miso, chili sauce, and garlic in a small bowl. Stir or whisk to make a smooth sauce. Pour over the pasta and toss until evenly coated. Garnish with the cilantro, green onions, and peanuts.

Per serving: 502 calories, 13 g protein, 14 g fat (2 g sat), 84 g carbs, 427 mg sodium, 19 mg calcium, 3 g fiber

wild rice and mushroom pilaf

MAKES 4 SERVINGS

Although this dish can be enjoyed year-round, it's especially satisfying in autumn and winter, as it's infused with the warming flavors associated with those cool-weather seasons. It can also be served as a side dish for eight and makes an impressive stuffing for baked winter squash.

1 cup brown and wild rice blend
2¼ cups no-salt-added gluten-free vegetable broth or water
1 tablespoon extra-virgin olive oil or coconut oil
1 large onion, chopped
3 stalks celery, diced
8 ounces mushrooms, sliced
2 cloves garlic, minced or pressed
1 tablespoon rubbed sage
1 teaspoon dried thyme
½ teaspoon sea salt
2 cups no-salt-added cooked or canned chickpeas, drained
½ cup dried cranberries
½ cup chopped flat-leaf parsley, lightly packed
½ cup chopped toasted pecans
Freshly ground black pepper

Put the rice in a large saucepan. Add the broth and bring to a boil over medium-high heat. Decrease the heat to low, cover, and simmer until the liquid is completely absorbed and the grains are tender, 45 to 50 minutes.

Put the oil in a large saucepan over medium heat. When hot, add the onion and celery and cook, stirring frequently, until tender, about 10 minutes. Add the mushrooms, garlic, sage, thyme, and salt and cook, stirring frequently, until the mushrooms are tender, 8 to 10 minutes. Add the chickpeas and cook, stirring frequently, until heated through, about 5 minutes. Add the cooked rice, cranberries, parsley, and pecans and toss gently to combine. Season with pepper to taste.

Per serving: 507 calories, 15 g protein, 17 g fat (2 g sat), 79 g carbs, 257 mg sodium, 84 mg calcium, 11 g fiber
Note: Analysis does not include freshly ground black pepper.

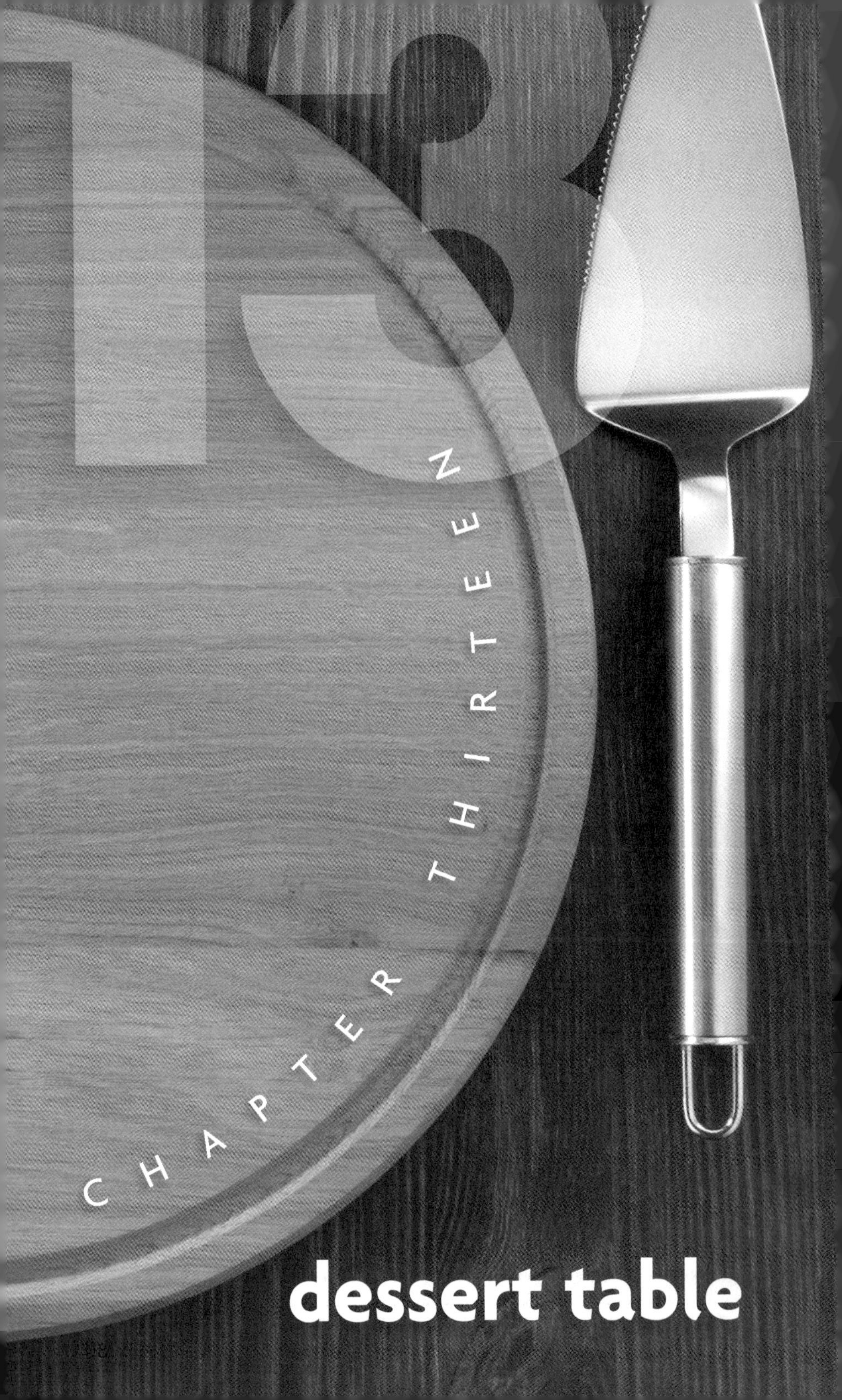

13

CHAPTER THIRTEEN

dessert table

chocolate sheet cake

This moist, light cake is perfect for any party, holiday, or special gathering. Serve it plain or spread with your favorite frosting.

2¾ cups GF All-Purpose Flour Mix (page 36) or other gluten-free all-purpose flour

⅔ cup unsweetened gluten-free cocoa powder

¼ cup quinoa flour

2 teaspoons baking soda

1¼ teaspoons xanthan gum

2 cups unbleached cane sugar

2 cups water

⅔ cup organic canola, safflower oil, or other neutral oil

2 teaspoons cider vinegar or freshly squeezed lemon juice

2 teaspoons gluten-free vanilla extract

Preheat the oven to 350 degrees F. Generously oil a 13 x 9-inch metal baking pan.

Put the flour mix, cocoa powder, quinoa flour, baking soda, and xanthan gum in a large bowl and whisk to combine.

Put the sugar, water, oil, vinegar, and vanilla extract in a separate large bowl. Using an electric mixer on medium speed, gradually beat in the flour mixture in three additions, beating well after each addition. Immediately pour into the oiled baking pan. Bake on the center rack of the oven for about 45 minutes, or until a toothpick inserted in the center tests clean. Let cool in the pan on a rack before serving. Cool completely before frosting.

Per serving: 318 calories, 3 g protein, 13 g fat (1 g sat), 49 g carbs, 233 mg sodium, 16 mg calcium, 5 g fiber

glazed lemon pound cake

This satisfying cake makes a wonderful dessert or special breakfast. Serve it with your favorite herbal tea and feel your cares melt away.

CAKE

⅓ cup coconut oil

1 cup unbleached cane sugar

2 tablespoons applesauce

2 teaspoons grated lemon zest

2¼ cups GF All-Purpose Flour Mix (page 36) or other gluten-free all-purpose flour

¼ cup quinoa flour

1 teaspoon xanthan gum

1 teaspoon gluten-free baking powder

½ teaspoon baking soda

¼ teaspoon sea salt

½ cup water

¼ cup freshly squeezed lemon juice

1 teaspoon gluten-free lemon extract

LEMON GLAZE

2 tablespoons unbleached cane sugar

2 tablespoons freshly squeezed lemon juice

Preheat the oven to 350 degrees F. Generously oil an 8½ x 4¼-inch metal loaf pan.

To make the cake, put the coconut oil and sugar in a large bowl and beat with an electric mixer on medium speed until light and fluffy. Add the applesauce and lemon zest and beat on low speed until blended.

Put the flour mix, quinoa flour, xanthan gum, baking powder, baking soda, and salt in a medium bowl and whisk to combine. Put the water, lemon juice, and lemon extract in a small bowl or measuring cup and stir to combine. With the mixer on medium speed, beat the dry ingredients into the sugar mixture, alternating with the lemon water and beginning and ending with the dry ingredients. Mix until just combined. Spoon the batter into the oiled loaf pan. The batter will be thick and somewhat elastic.

Bake on the center rack of the oven for about 60 minutes, until the top is golden brown and a toothpick inserted in the center tests clean. Cool the cake in the pan on a rack for 5 minutes, then remove from pan and cool on the rack.

To make the glaze, put the sugar and lemon juice in a small saucepan. Bring to a boil over medium-high heat and boil for 1 minute. Remove from the heat and let cool. Put a sheet of waxed paper under the cake and rack. Drizzle the glaze over the cake while the glaze and cake are still a little warm.

GLAZED LEMON–POPPY SEED POUND CAKE: Beat ¼ cup of poppy seeds into the batter before spooning it into the pan.

GLAZED LEMON–SESAME SEED POUND CAKE: Beat ¼ cup of toasted sesame seeds into the batter before spooning it into the pan.

GLAZED ORANGE POUND CAKE: Replace the lemon zest with an equal amount of orange zest, replace the lemon juice with an equal amount of freshly squeezed orange juice, and replace the lemon extract with gluten-free orange extract. This version may be combined with either of the seed variations above.

Per serving: 241 calories, 3 g protein, 8 g fat (6 g sat), 42 g carbs, 141 mg sodium, 19 mg calcium, 3 g fiber

basic two-layer white cake

Light, fluffy, and moist, this divine cake is ideal for every special occasion. Spread your favorite filling or fruit jam between the layers and frost the top and sides. A delicious combination is a fruit-jam filling between the layers and vanilla frosting on the top and sides.

6 tablespoons coconut oil

1½ cups unbleached cane sugar

¼ cup applesauce

1½ tablespoons grated lemon zest

2¾ cups GF All-Purpose Flour Mix (page 36) or other gluten-free all-purpose flour

¼ cup quinoa flour

1¼ teaspoons xanthan gum

1½ teaspoons gluten-free baking powder

¾ teaspoon baking soda

¼ teaspoon sea salt

1 cup plus 2 tablespoons water

1½ tablespoons freshly squeezed lemon juice

1½ teaspoons gluten-free vanilla extract

Preheat the oven to 350 degrees F. Generously oil two nonstick 9-inch round metal cake pans. Line the bottom of the cake pans with parchment paper. Use the pan to trace a circle on the parchment paper and then cut it to fit the bottom of the pan.

Put the coconut oil and sugar in a large bowl and beat with an electric mixer on medium speed until light and fluffy. With the mixer on low speed, beat in the applesauce and lemon zest.

Put flour mix, quinoa flour, xanthan gum, baking powder, baking soda, and salt in a medium bowl and whisk to combine. Put the water, lemon juice, and vanilla extract in a separate medium bowl and whisk to combine. With the mixer on low speed, beat the dry ingredients into the sugar mixture, alternating with the lemon water and beginning and ending with the dry ingredients. Mix until just combined. The batter will be thick and somewhat elastic. Spoon the batter into the prepared pans and smooth the tops.

Bake for 20 to 25 minutes, until the tops are golden brown and a toothpick inserted in the center of each cake tests clean. Cool the cakes in the pans on two racks for 5 minutes, then remove from the pans and cool on the racks. Cool completely before frosting.

Per serving: 290 calories, 3 g protein, 10 g fat (7 g sat), 51 g carbs, 125 mg sodium, 15 mg calcium, 3 g fiber

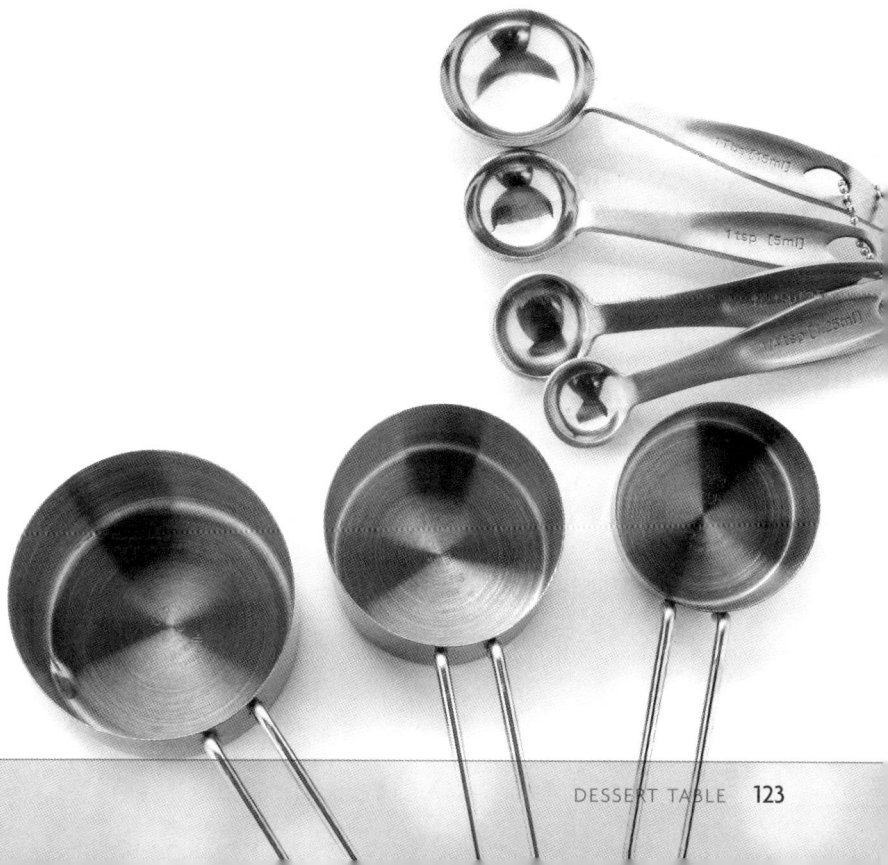

basic three-layer white cake

Multilayer cakes make for spectacular presentations and are especially well suited for celebrations and major life events, such as weddings, graduations, and anniversaries. Fill the layers and frost the top and sides with your favorite frosting, and don't skimp on the gluten-free decorations, including edible flowers.

9 tablespoons coconut oil

2¼ cups unbleached cane sugar

6 tablespoons applesauce

2 tablespoons grated lemon zest

4½ cups GF All-Purpose Flour Mix (page 36) or other gluten-free all-purpose flour

⅓ cup quinoa flour

2 teaspoons xanthan gum

2¼ teaspoons gluten-free baking powder

1 teaspoon baking soda

¼ teaspoon plus a pinch sea salt

1⅔ cups water

2½ tablespoons freshly squeezed lemon juice

2½ teaspoons gluten-free vanilla extract

Preheat the oven to 350 degrees F. Generously oil three nonstick 9-inch round metal cake pans. Line the bottom of the cake pans with parchment paper. Use the pan to trace a circle on the parchment paper and then cut it to fit the bottom of the pan.

Put the coconut oil and sugar in a large bowl and beat with an electric mixer on medium speed until light and fluffy. With the mixer on low speed, beat in the applesauce and lemon zest.

Put flour mix, quinoa flour, xanthan gum, baking powder, baking soda, and salt in a medium bowl and whisk to combine. Put the water, lemon juice, and vanilla extract in a separate medium bowl and whisk to combine. With the mixer on low speed, beat the dry ingredients into the sugar mixture, alternating with the lemon water and beginning and ending with the dry ingredients. Mix until just combined. The batter will be thick and somewhat elastic. Spoon the batter into the prepared pans and smooth the tops.

Bake for 20 to 25 minutes, until the tops are golden brown and a toothpick inserted in the center of each cake tests clean. Cool the cakes in the pans for 5 minutes, then remove from the pans and cool on racks. Cool completely before frosting.

Per serving: 302 calories, 3 g protein, 10 g fat (7 g sat), 51 g carbs, 125 mg sodium, 15 mg calcium, 3 g fiber

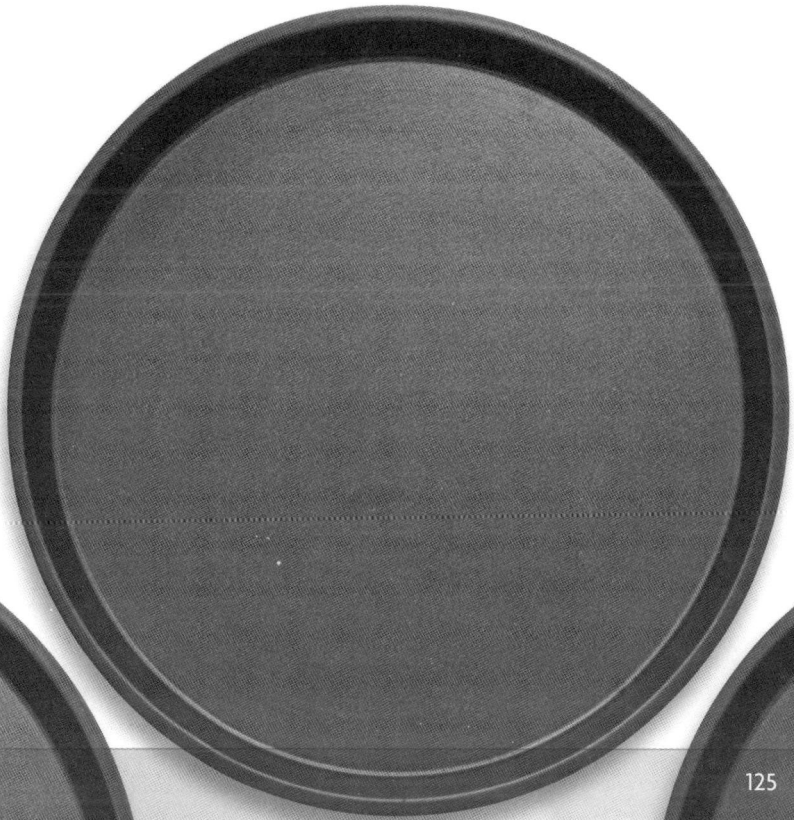

chocolate snack cake

This cake is light and divinely chocolatey. Its small dimensions make it ideal for snack-sized portions.

1¼ cups GF All-Purpose Flour Mix (page 36) or other gluten-free all-purpose flour

½ cup unsweetened gluten-free cocoa powder

1 teaspoon baking soda

¾ teaspoon xanthan gum

½ teaspoon sea salt

1 cup light brown sugar, firmly packed

½ cup organic canola oil or other neutral oil

2 teaspoons gluten-free vanilla extract

¼ cup applesauce

¼ cup pure maple syrup

¼ cup gluten-free plain or vanilla nondairy milk or water

Preheat the oven to 350 degrees F. Generously oil a 9-inch round or 8-inch square metal cake pan.

Put the flour mix, cocoa powder, baking soda, xanthan gum, and salt in a large bowl and whisk to combine.

Put the sugar, oil, and vanilla extract in a separate large bowl and beat with an electric mixer on low speed to combine. Beat in the applesauce and maple syrup. Then beat in the milk with the mixer on low speed. Gradually add the flour mixture in three additions, beating well after each addition. Pour into the oiled cake pan and bake for 30 minutes, or until a toothpick inserted in the center tests clean. Let cool in the pan on a rack before serving. Cool completely before frosting.

Per serving: 339 calories, 2 g protein, 15 g fat (1 g sat), 54 g carbs, 275 mg sodium, 34 mg calcium, 2 g fiber

chocolate–peanut butter pie

MAKES 1 PIE, 10 SERVINGS

This luxurious chocolate pie is creamy and rich but contains no dairy products or gluten. In fact, it doesn't even involve any baking!

1 cup ground or very finely chopped walnuts (see tip)
2½ cups gluten-free chocolate chips
3 very ripe bananas, broken into chunks
1 cup smooth peanut butter
½ cup coconut cream (see tip)
1 teaspoon gluten-free vanilla extract

Sprinkle ½ cup of the walnuts over the bottom of an 8-inch pie pan or 8-inch round cake pan.

Put the chocolate chips in the top of a double boiler and heat over simmering water, stirring occasionally, until the chocolate is just melted. If you don't have a double boiler, use a large saucepan directly over low heat, stirring almost constantly to prevent burning, or use a microwave. Put the melted chocolate, bananas, peanut butter, coconut cream, and vanilla extract in a food processor and process until smooth and creamy. Pour evenly over the walnuts and smooth the top. Sprinkle the remaining walnuts around the rim of the pie filling to create a decorative border.

Put in the freezer until firm, about 3 hours, before serving. Serve chilled. Store in the freezer.

TIPS

- Take care not to overprocess the walnuts when grinding them or you'll end up with walnut butter.
- For the coconut cream, refrigerate an unopened can of coconut milk, keeping it upright in the refrigerator. When the coconut milk is chilled, the cream will rise to the top. Open the upright can and spoon off the cream.

Per serving: 569 calories, 16 g protein, 51 g fat (18 g sat), 45 g carbs, 119 mg sodium, 112 mg calcium, 7 g fiber

super-fudgy brownies

These are the ultimate fudge brownies. No one will believe they're made without eggs or dairy products, let alone that they're gluten-free.

1 cup unbleached cane sugar

½ cup pure maple syrup

½ cup organic canola oil, safflower oil, or other neutral oil

⅓ cup applesauce

1 teaspoon gluten-free vanilla extract

1 cup GF All-Purpose Flour Mix (page 36) or other gluten-free all-purpose flour

½ cup unsweetened gluten-free cocoa powder

2 teaspoons gluten-free baking powder

½ teaspoon xanthan gum

¼ teaspoon sea salt

½ cup chopped walnuts (optional)

Preheat the oven to 350 degrees F. Oil an 8-inch square metal baking pan.

Put the sugar, maple syrup, oil, applesauce, and vanilla extract in a large bowl and stir to combine.

Put the flour mix, cocoa powder, baking powder, xanthan gum, and salt in a medium bowl and whisk to combine. Gradually add to the oil mixture in three additions, stirring until well blended after each addition. Stir in the walnuts if using.

Spread the batter evenly into the oiled baking pan. Shake the pan so the batter reaches all corners equally. Bake on the center rack of the oven for 40 to 45 minutes, or until a toothpick inserted in the center tests clean. Cool in the pan on a rack. Cool completely before cutting into squares (see tip).

TIP: The texture of these brownies is even better a day or two after baking. If you cannot wait that long, be sure to let them cool *completely* before cutting, as this will prevent them from being gummy or falling apart.

DECADENT DOUBLE-FUDGE BROWNIES: Stir ¼ cup of gluten-free mini chocolate chips into the batter before pouring into the oiled pan.

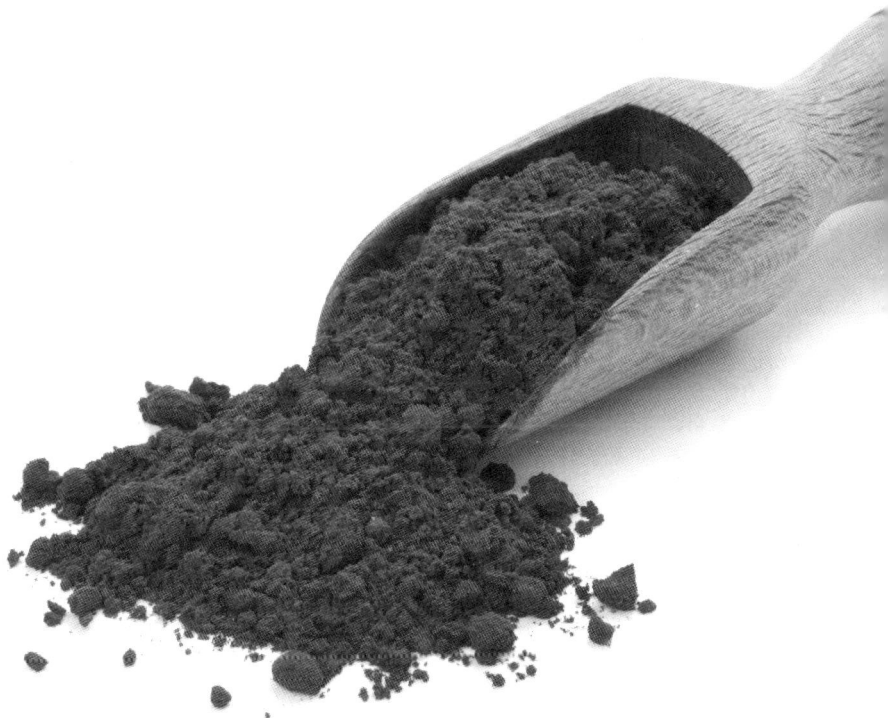

Per brownie: 152 calories, 1 g protein, 7 g fat (1 g sat), 22 g carbs, 70 mg sodium, 14 mg calcium, 1 g fiber

blueberry streusel coffee cake

MAKES 1 CAKE, 10 SERVINGS

Packed with fruit and topped with a sweet crumble, this wholesome, moist coffee cake is fabulous for breakfast, brunch, or dessert. Because the recipe calls for frozen blueberries, it can be made year-round. Don't thaw the berries beforehand.

CAKE

¾ cup unbleached cane sugar

¼ cup soft coconut oil

2 tablespoons applesauce

½ teaspoon gluten-free vanilla extract

1¾ cups GF All-Purpose Flour Mix (page 36) or other gluten-free all-purpose flour

¼ cup quinoa flour

2 teaspoons gluten-free baking powder

1 teaspoon xanthan gum

½ teaspoon sea salt

½ cup gluten-free plain or vanilla nondairy milk, lite coconut milk, or water

2 cups frozen blueberries (see tip)

TOPPING

½ cup unbleached cane sugar

⅓ cup GF All-Purpose Flour Mix (page 36) or other gluten-free all-purpose flour

3 tablespoons soft coconut oil

½ teaspoon ground cinnamon

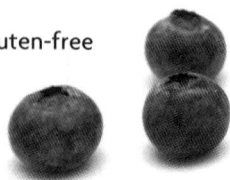

Preheat the oven to 375 degrees F. Generously oil a 9-inch square metal baking pan or 9-inch round metal cake pan.

To make the cake, put the sugar, oil, applesauce, and vanilla extract in a large bowl and stir to combine. Put the flour mix, quinoa flour, baking powder, xanthan gum, and salt in a medium bowl and whisk to combine. Add half the flour mixture to the sugar mixture and beat with an electric mixer on medium speed to incorporate. Beat in the milk, then beat in the rest of the flour mixture. Mix until just combined. Fold in the blueberries. Spoon the batter into the oiled baking pan.

To make the topping, put sugar, flour mix, oil, and cinnamon in a medium bowl and stir with a fork until evenly blended and crumbly. Sprinkle over the batter. Bake for 1 hour, or until the top starts to brown and a toothpick inserted in the center tests clean. Cool in the pan on a rack before serving.

TIP: If you prefer to use fresh blueberries, decrease the baking time to 45 minutes.

VARIATION: Add ½ cup of chopped pecans to the topping mixture before sprinkling over the batter.

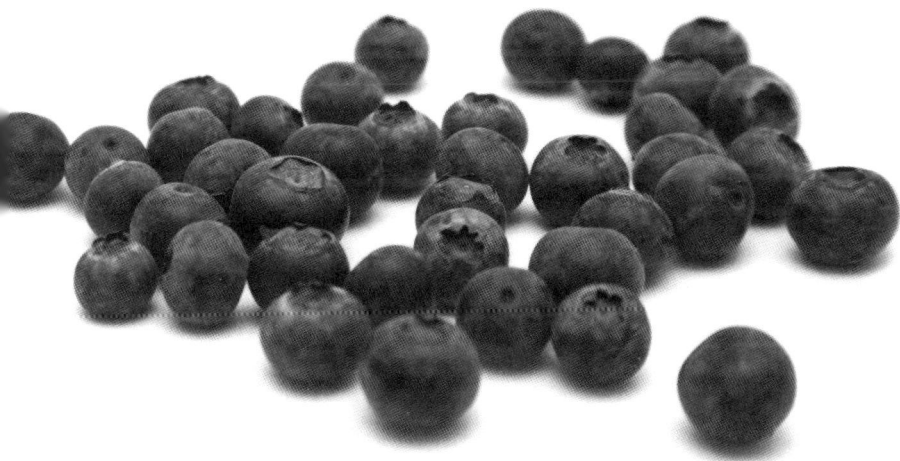

Per serving: 229 calories, 3 g protein, 7 g fat (5 g sat), 455 g carbs, 110 mg sodium, 11 mg calcium, 3 g fiber

heavenly date squares

These popular squares have a delectable layer of date butter sandwiched between a thick, melt-in-your-mouth shortbread crust. One bite and your taste buds will be in heaven.

FILLING

1½ cups chopped dates, packed

¾ cup water

¼ teaspoon sea salt

CRUST

3 cups GF All-Purpose Flour Mix (page 36) or other gluten-free all-purpose flour

⅔ cup unbleached cane sugar

1½ teaspoons xanthan gum

¾ teaspoon ground cinnamon

½ teaspoon gluten-free baking powder

½ teaspoon baking soda

¼ teaspoon sea salt

¼ cup organic canola or safflower oil

¼ cup soft coconut oil

Preheat the oven to 350 degrees F.

To make the filling, put the dates, water, and salt in a medium saucepan and bring to a boil over high heat. Decrease the heat to medium-low, cover, and simmer, stirring once or twice, until very soft, about 15 minutes. Remove from the heat and let rest, covered, until cool.

To make the crust, put the flour mix, sugar, xanthan gum, cinnamon, baking powder, baking soda, and salt in a large bowl and whisk to combine. Stir in the canola oil and coconut oil with a fork, then finish by working them in with your hands until well combined.

Press half the crust mixture into the bottom of an unoiled 8-inch square metal baking pan. The dough will be crumbly, so press it firmly into the pan. Carefully spread the date mixture evenly over the crust, spreading it out with the back of a large spoon. Crumble the remaining crust mixture evenly over the date mixture to form a top crust. Pat it down firmly but gently. Bake for about 50 minutes, until the top is lightly browned. Let cool in the pan on a rack. Cut into squares while warm. The crust will be very crumbly when hot. As the squares cool, the crust will become firmer.

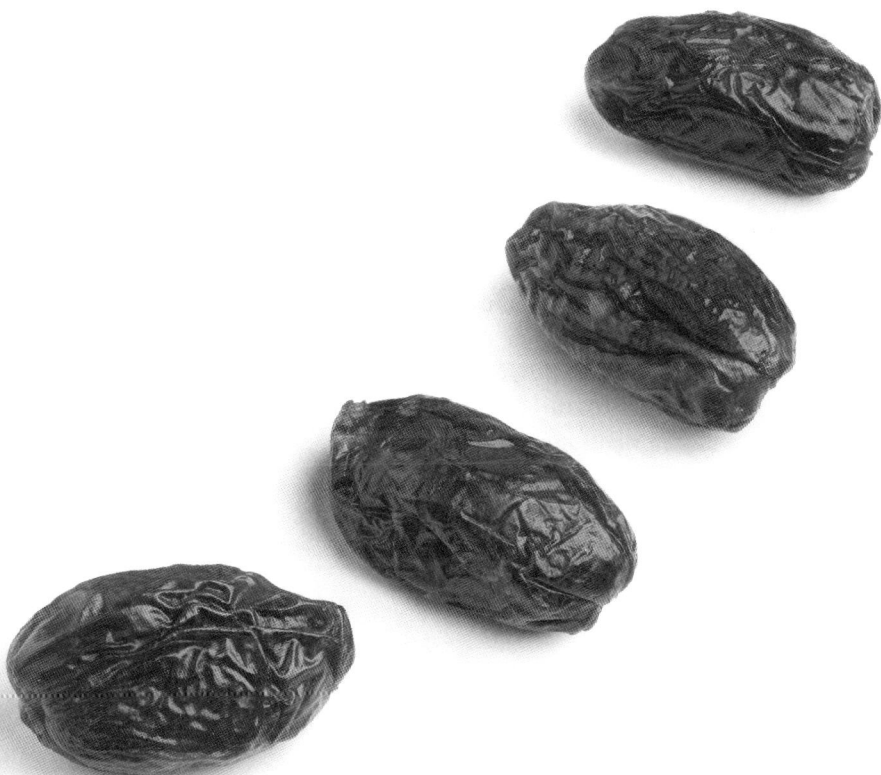

Per square: 223 calories, 3 g protein, 8 g fat (3 g sat), 24 g carbs, 104 mg sodium, 16 mg calcium, 3 g fiber

apricot squares

These scrumptious treats are light and crumbly, perfect as a midday snack with a cup of ginger tea.

2¾ cups GF All-Purpose Flour Mix (page 36) or other gluten-free all-purpose flour

¼ cup quinoa flour

2 teaspoons ground cinnamon

1¼ teaspoons xanthan gum

¾ cup soft coconut oil

1 cup light brown sugar, firmly packed

1 teaspoon gluten-free vanilla extract

1 cup chopped dried apricots

1 cup coarsely chopped walnuts, sunflower seeds, or pumpkin seeds

Preheat the oven to 350 degrees F. Oil a 13 x 9-inch metal baking pan.

Put the flour mix, quinoa flour, cinnamon, and xanthan gum in a medium bowl and whisk to combine. Put the coconut oil, brown sugar, and vanilla extract in a large bowl and beat with an electric mixer on medium speed until light and fluffy. Gradually beat in the dry ingredients in three additions. The mixture will resemble coarse crumbs. Stir in the apricots and walnuts.

Pat firmly into the oiled baking pan. Bake on the center rack for 40 to 45 minutes, until the top is golden. Cool completely in the pan on a rack before cutting into squares.

Per square: 158 calories, 3 g protein, 9 g fat (6 g sat), 15 g carbs, 2 mg sodium, 12 mg calcium, 3 g fiber

divine macaroons

Stored in a tightly sealed tin at room temperature, these cookies will retain their moist, chewy texture for a week.

2½ cups unsweetened shredded dried coconut

½ cup GF All-Purpose Flour Mix (page 36) or other gluten-free all-purpose flour

½ teaspoon xanthan gum

¼ teaspoon sea salt

½ cup water

½ cup pure maple syrup

1 teaspoon gluten-free almond, orange, lemon, coconut, or vanilla extract

Preheat the oven to 325 degrees F. Line a baking sheet with parchment paper or a silicone baking mat.

Put the coconut, flour mix, xanthan gum, and salt in a large bowl and whisk to combine. Put the water, maple syrup, and almond extract in a small bowl and stir to combine. Pour into the dry ingredients and stir until evenly blended.

Using moistened fingers, form into 1½-inch balls, pressing the mixture together firmly. Put the balls on the lined baking sheet as they are formed. Bake on the center rack of the oven for 30 to 35 minutes, until golden brown. Let cool completely before serving.

CHOCOLATE-TOPPED MACAROONS: Melt ½ cup of chopped gluten-free dark chocolate in a double boiler or microwave. Drizzle over the cooled macaroons.

Per macaroon: 168 calories, 1 g protein, 11 g fat (10 g sat), 4 g carbs, 35 mg sodium, 8 mg calcium, 3 g fiber

chocolate chippers

These magnificent cookies are exceptionally chocolaty, which is the only way a chocolate chip cookie worthy of its name ought to be. Cool these little treasures completely before storing or eating them.

- 1½ cups GF All-Purpose Flour Mix (page 36) or other gluten-free all-purpose flour
- ½ teaspoon baking soda
- ½ teaspoon xanthan gum
- ¼ teaspoon sea salt
- ¾ cup light brown sugar, firmly packed
- ⅓ cup unbleached cane sugar
- ¼ cup organic canola or safflower oil
- 2 tablespoons applesauce
- 2 teaspoons gluten-free vanilla extract
- 1½ cups gluten-free chocolate chips

Preheat the oven to 350 degrees F. Line two baking sheets with parchment paper or silicone baking mats.

Put the flour mix, baking soda, xanthan gum, and salt in a medium bowl and whisk to combine. Put the brown sugar, cane sugar, oil, applesauce, and vanilla extract in a large bowl and beat with an electric mixer on medium speed until light and fluffy. With the mixer on low speed, gradually beat in the flour mixture in three additions. The dough will be very stiff and sticky.

Stir in the chocolate chips, using your hands if necessary. Drop by slightly rounded tablespoons onto the lined baking sheets, keeping the cookies an inch or two apart to allow them to spread. Bake on the center rack of the oven, one sheet at time, for 12 to 15 minutes, or until the cookies are lightly browned. Let cool on the baking sheets for a full 5 minutes, then transfer to racks using a metal spatula to finish cooling completely.

NUTTY CHOCOLATE CHIPPERS: Decrease the amount of chocolate chips to 1 cup and add ½ cup of coarsely chopped walnuts, pecans, peanuts, sunflower seeds, or pumpkin seeds.

Per cookie: 131 calories, 1 g protein, 7 g fat (3 g sat), 17 g carbs, 46 mg sodium, 20 mg calcium, 1 g fiber

crispy maple-vanilla wafers

These delectable, wafer-thin cookies are a delightful treat. For special occasions, sprinkle the tops lightly with colored sugar just before baking, or gently press in gluten-free chocolate or multicolored jimmies, shredded dried coconut, mini chocolate chips, or your favorite cookie decorations.

> 1½ cups GF All-Purpose Flour Mix (page 36) or other gluten-free all-purpose flour mix
> ½ teaspoon gluten-free baking powder
> ½ teaspoon xanthan gum
> ⅛ teaspoon sea salt
> ¼ cup pure maple syrup
> 3 tablespoons organic canola or safflower oil
> 1 tablespoon gluten-free vanilla extract

Preheat the oven to 350 degrees F. Line two baking sheets with parchment paper or silicone baking mats.

Put the flour mix, baking powder, xanthan gum, and salt in a large bowl and whisk to combine. Put the maple syrup, oil, and vanilla extract in a small bowl and whisk to combine. Pour into the dry ingredients and stir until well combined.

Using your hands, form into balls, each about the size of a walnut. Put the balls an inch or two apart on the lined baking sheets. Press each ball into a thin disk using the bottom of a large, heavy jar or drinking glass. (Be sure the bottom is perfectly flat or it will leave an imprint in the cookies.) To lift the jar or glass from the cookie, turn it slightly before lifting. The dough should be very thin, about ¼ inch thick or a little less.

Bake on the center rack of the oven, one sheet at a time, for about 12 minutes, or until the edges and bottoms of the cookies are golden brown. Let cool on the baking sheets. Cool completely before storing.

Per wafer: 70 calories, 1 g protein, 2 g fat (0.2 g sat), 3 g carbs, 28 mg sodium, 5 mg calcium, 1 g fiber

chocolate crinkles

The tops of these cookies crinkle, or crack, when baked, creating an attractive contrast between the dark chocolate cookie and the white confectioners' sugar on top. With a deep chocolate flavor reminiscent of brownies, they are as delicious as they are attractive. The cookies will firm up as they cool, so be careful not to overbake them or they will become too hard.

1¼ cups GF All-Purpose Flour Mix (page 36) or other gluten-free all-purpose flour

¼ cup unsweetened gluten-free cocoa powder

3 tablespoons quinoa flour

1 tablespoon chickpea flour

1 teaspoon gluten-free baking powder

¼ teaspoon sea salt

¼ cup soft coconut oil

1 cup unbleached cane sugar

1 teaspoon gluten-free vanilla extract

2 tablespoons applesauce

1 tablespoon cold water

¼ cup gluten-free confectioners' sugar

Preheat the oven to 325 degrees F. Line two or three baking sheets with parchment paper or silicone baking mats.

Put the flour mix, cocoa powder, quinoa flour, chickpea flour, baking powder, and salt in a medium bowl and whisk to combine. Put the oil, sugar, and vanilla extract in a large bowl and beat with an electric mixer on medium speed until light and fluffy. Beat in the applesauce and water.

Gradually beat in the dry ingredients in three additions. The dough will be stiff. Put the confectioners' sugar on a plate. Using your hands, roll the dough into 1-inch balls, then roll the balls in the confectioners' sugar. Put the balls on the lined baking sheets as they are made, arranging them two inches apart. Bake on the center rack of the oven, one sheet at a time, for 16 minutes. Do not overbake. Let cool on the baking sheets for a full 5 minutes, then transfer to racks using a metal spatula to finish cooling completely.

Per cookie: 50 calories, 0 g protein, 2 g fat (1 g sat), 8 g carbs, 21 mg sodium, 3 mg calcium, 0 g fiber

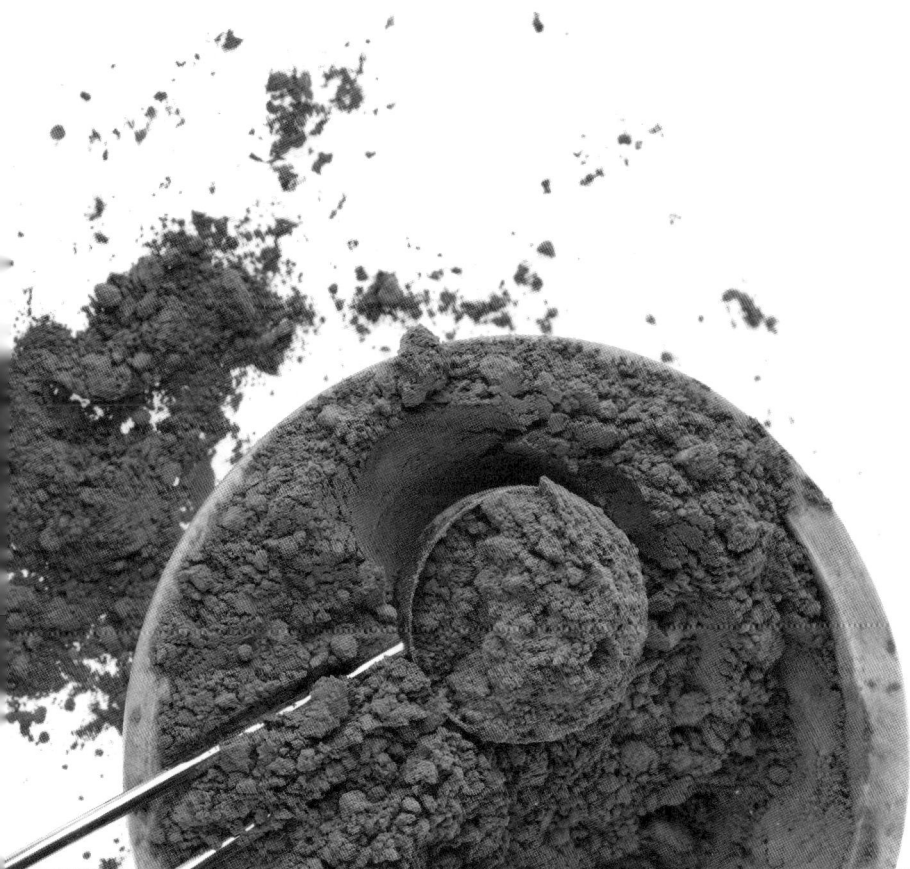

flourless
chocolate shortbread cookies

These amazing shortbread cookies use almond flour rather than grain flour to create a crispy, buttery treat. You won't believe how simple, quick, and decadent tasting they are.

- ¾ cup plus 2 tablespoons almond flour
- 3 tablespoons gluten-free vegan butter, at room temperature
- 3 tablespoons gluten-free confectioners' sugar
- 2 tablespoons unsweetened gluten-free cocoa powder
- ½ teaspoon gluten-free vanilla extract
- ⅛ teaspoon sea salt
- ⅓ cup chopped walnuts or pecans

Put the almond flour, butter, sugar, cocoa powder, vanilla extract, and salt in a large bowl. Beat with an electric mixer on low speed until a dough forms. Alternatively, mix the ingredients by hand using a wooden spoon until a dough forms. Stir in the walnuts until evenly distributed.

Put a large piece of plastic wrap on a flat surface. Transfer the dough to the plastic wrap and shape into a 7 x 2-inch log. Wrap the plastic around the dough and shape into a log again if necessary. Refrigerate until chilled and firm, 1 to 2 hours.

When you're ready to bake the cookies, preheat the oven to 350 degrees F. Line a baking sheet with parchment paper or a silicone baking mat.

Unwrap the cookie dough and slice into ¼-inch-thick rounds using a sharp knife. Arrange the rounds on the lined baking sheet and bake for 12 to 14 minutes, until the cookies just start to brown. Remove from the oven and let cool on the baking sheet for 10 minutes, then transfer to racks using a metal spatula to finish cooling completely.

Per cookie: 74 calories, 2 g protein, 6 g fat (1 g sat), 4 g carbs, 35 mg sodium, 20 mg calcium, 1 g fiber

crunchy peanut cookies

These cookies have very few ingredients, so as long as your pantry is stocked, you can whip them up whenever the urge strikes. They store well when kept in a sealed tin at room temperature, and they're so filling and nutritious you can just grab some for an on-the-go breakfast or an energizing snack.

6 tablespoons smooth or chunky peanut butter

6 tablespoons pure maple syrup

½ cup coarsely chopped gluten-free unsalted dry-roasted peanuts

¼ teaspoon ground cinnamon (optional)

⅛ teaspoon ground cardamom (optional)

⅛ teaspoon ground nutmeg (optional)

1 cup gluten-free crispy rice cereal

Preheat the oven to 350 degrees F. Line a baking sheet with parchment paper or a silicone baking mat.

Put the peanut butter and maple syrup in a medium bowl and stir until well blended. Add the peanuts and the optional cinnamon, cardamom, and nutmeg and stir until well combined. Gently fold in the cereal until evenly distributed.

Using your hands, form into 20 small balls and put them on the lined baking sheet as they are made. Flatten each ball slightly with your hand. Bake for 12 to 15 minutes, until the edges are golden. Transfer to racks to cool.

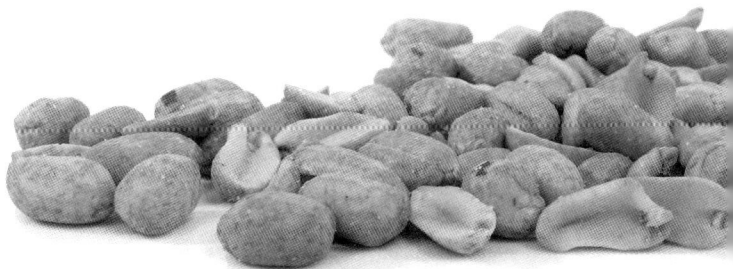

Per cookie: 66 calories, 2 g protein, 4 g fat (1 g sat), 7 g carbs, 36 mg sodium, 6 mg calcium, 1 g fiber

coconut cookie-dough balls

These no-bake treats are so simple to pull together and are sure to satisfy even the most die-hard sweet tooth.

1 cup gluten-free rolled oats

1 ripe banana, sliced

½ cup unsweetened shredded dried coconut

3 tablespoons pure maple syrup

2 tablespoons soft coconut oil

1 teaspoon gluten-free vanilla extract

½ cup gluten-free chocolate chips

Put the oats in a food processor and pulse until coarsely chopped. Add the banana, coconut, maple syrup, oil, and vanilla extract and pulse until just combined, stopping once or twice as needed to scrape down the work bowl. Transfer to a medium bowl and stir in the chocolate chips. Cover and refrigerate for 10 minutes.

Remove from the refrigerator and form into 12 balls. Serve immediately or transfer to a sealed container and store in the refrigerator.

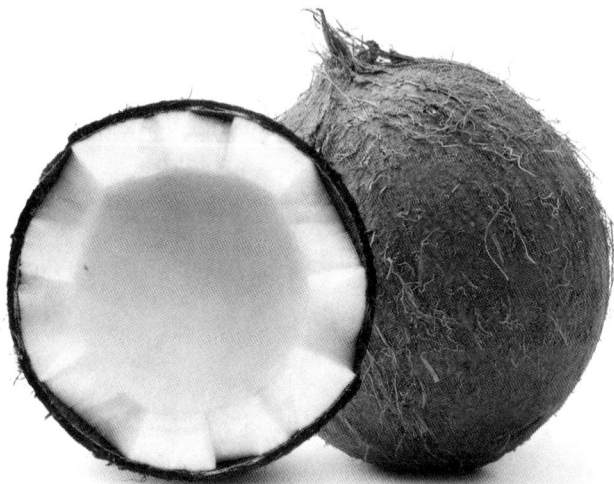

Per ball: 139 calories, 2 g protein, 8 g fat (6 g sat), 16 g carbs, 2 mg sodium, 22 mg calcium, 2 g fiber

cookie-dough nibbles

These no-bake nuggets are irresistibly addictive. They make a sweet, satisfying treat any time of day or night.

⅓ cup coconut flour

¼ cup almond flour

Pinch sea salt

¾ cup almond butter or other nut butter

⅓ cup pure maple syrup

¼ teaspoon gluten-free vanilla extract

¼ cup gluten-free mini or regular chocolate chips

2 tablespoons chopped walnuts or pecans or additional chocolate chips

Put the coconut flour, almond flour, and salt in a medium bowl and whisk to combine. Add the almond butter, maple syrup, and vanilla extract and stir until smooth and well combined. Add the chocolate chips and walnuts and stir until evenly distributed. Form into 24 bite-sized balls. Transfer to a storage container and put in the freezer for 30 minutes before serving. Store in the refrigerator.

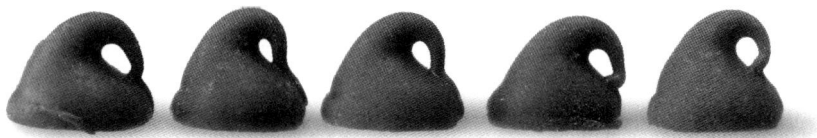

Per nibble: 88 calories, 3 g protein, 6 g fat (1 g sat), 7 g carbs, 34 mg sodium, 59 mg calcium, 2 g fiber

puffy bars

Sweet and quick, this recipe is a real crowd-pleaser.

> 8 cups gluten-free puffed rice cereal
> 1 cup light brown sugar, firmly packed
> ½ cup gluten-free brown rice syrup
> ⅓ cup organic canola or safflower oil
> ¼ cup unsweetened gluten-free cocoa powder
> 1 teaspoon gluten-free vanilla extract

Put the cereal in a large bowl. Put the brown sugar, rice syrup, oil, and cocoa powder in a medium saucepan and bring to a boil over medium-high heat. Boil for 1 minute, stirring constantly. Remove from the heat and stir in the vanilla extract. Pour over the cereal and mix well. Spread evenly into a 13 x 9-inch baking pan and let cool. Cut into bars or squares. Cool completely before storing. Store in a sealed container at room temperature.

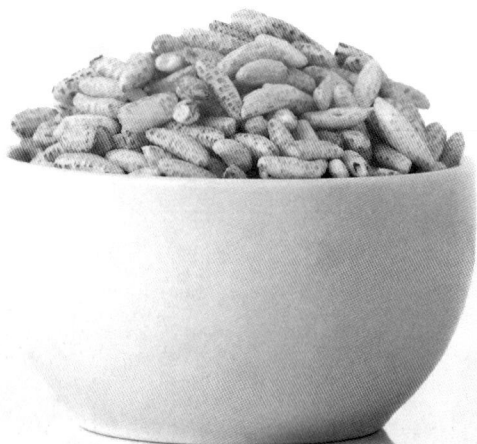

Per large bar: 149 calories, 1 g protein, 5 g fat (1 g sat), 26 g carbs, 133 mg sodium, 2 mg calcium, 1 g fiber

crispy rice bars

These rich, crunchy squares make a delicious dessert or sweet snack.

2 cups gluten-free crispy rice cereal

½ cup gluten-free chocolate chips, chopped walnuts or almonds, currants, raisins, or finely chopped dried apricots

⅔ cup gluten-free brown rice syrup

¼ cup tahini or almond butter

½ teaspoon gluten-free vanilla extract

Oil an 8-inch square baking pan or mist it with cooking spray.

Put the cereal and chocolate chips in a large bowl. Put the rice syrup and tahini in a small saucepan and warm over low heat, stirring occasionally, until the mixture is softened and smooth, about 5 minutes. Remove from the heat and stir in the vanilla extract. Let cool slightly, just until warm. Pour over the cereal mixture and stir gently. Work as quickly as possible so the chocolate chips don't melt. Pack the mixture evenly into the oiled baking pan, pressing gently with your fingers. Cover the pan with plastic wrap and chill in the refrigerator until firm, 1 to 2 hours. Cut into squares and store in a sealed container in the refrigerator.

Per square: 128 calories, 2 g protein, 5 g fat (2 g sat), 19 g carbs, 41 mg sodium, 15 mg calcium, 1 g fiber

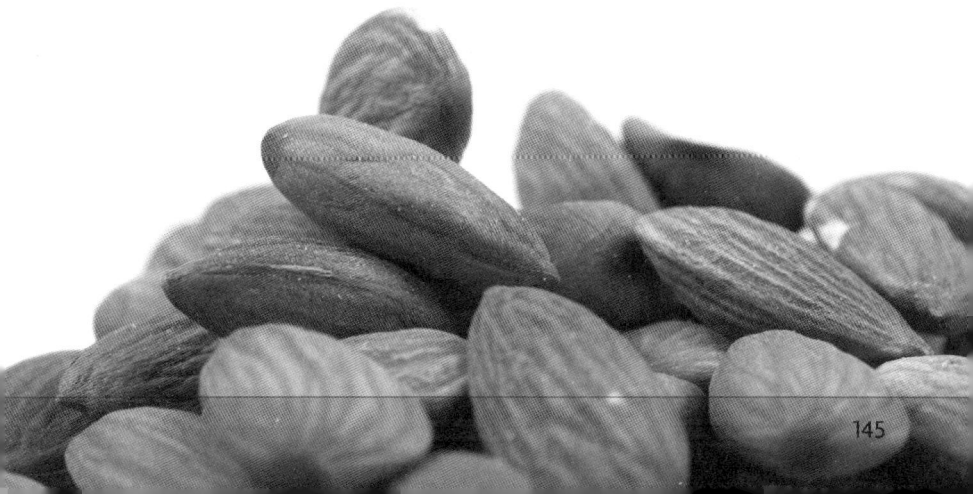

choco-currant cranberry squares

This simple combination of dried fruit, chocolate, and cereal can be stirred together in minutes.

½ cup pure maple syrup
¼ cup tahini or almond butter
2½ squares gluten-free semisweet baking chocolate
⅔ cup dried currants, dried cranberries, or a combination
1¼ cups gluten-free puffed rice cereal
1¼ cups gluten-free flaked cereal

Lightly oil an 8 x 4-inch loaf pan.

Put the maple syrup, tahini, and chocolate in the top of a double boiler and heat over boiling water, stirring occasionally, until the chocolate is just melted. If you don't have a double boiler, use a large saucepan directly over low heat, stirring almost constantly to prevent burning, or use a microwave. Remove from the heat and add the currants, puffed rice cereal, and flaked cereal. Stir until the chocolate mixture is evenly distributed. Press into the prepared loaf pan. Put in the refrigerator or freezer for 30 minutes to set. Cut into 10 squares. Store in a sealed container at room temperature or in the refrigerator.

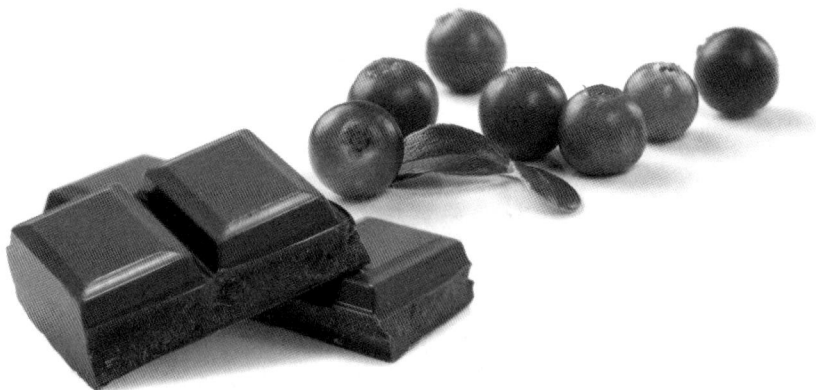

Per square: 159 calories, 3 g protein, 5 g fat (1 g sat), 26 g carbs, 67 mg sodium, 27 mg calcium, 2 g fiber

SUPPLIERS

The following online retailers provide a broad range of certified gluten-free products and ingredients to make your move to a gluten-free lifestyle enjoyable, safe, and delicious:

Enjoy Life: enjoylifefoods.com

Flavorganics: flavorganics.com

Free from Gluten: freefromgluten.com

Gluten Free Supermarket: glutenfree-supermarket.com

Gluten-Free Mall: glutenfreemall.com

GlutenFreePalace.com: glutenfreepalace.com

GlutenSolutions.com: glutensolutions.com

Penzeys: penzeys.com
(The company states that all their herbs and spices are gluten-free; however, their soup bases aren't vegan and aren't gluten-free.)

The Gluten Free Shoppe: theglutenfreeshoppe.com

Further Information

The following organizations will provide information and support as you embark on you gluten-free journey:

American Celiac Disease Alliance: americanceliac.org

Celiac Disease Foundation: celiac.org

Celiac Travel: celiactravel.com

Celiac.com: celiac.com

GlutenFree.com: glutenfree.com

National Foundation for Celiac Awareness: celiaccentral.org

National Institutes of Health Celiac Disease Awareness Campaign: celiac.nih.gov

INDEX

Recipe titles appear in *italics*.

A

abdominal pain, 2, 5
Africa, foods from, 21, 24
allergens/allergies, 6, 11, 12
All-Purpose Flour Mix, GF, 36
All-Purpose Herb Blend, 46
almond flour, 11, 32
alternatives to gluten-containing foods, 20
amaranth
  about, 22
  amaranth flour, 32
  amaranth pasta, 20
  in ancient civilizations, 21, 66
  Breakfast Cereal, 67
  cooking time for, 26
  as gluten-free, 11
  Quinoa, and Polenta Porridge, 65
amino acids, 5
Andes Mountains, quinoa grown in, 21, 23
anemia, 2
antibiotics as affecting "bad" bacteria, 6
antioxidants, in whole grains, 21
anxiety, 2, 3
Apricot Dressing, Curried Rice and Fruit Salad with, 79
Apricot Squares, 134
Arabian peninsula, sorghum from, 24
arborio rice, 24
arrowroot starch, 11, 20, 32
Asia, sorghum from, 24
Asian rice noodles, 20
autoimmunity/autoimmune disorders, 2, 6

B

B vitamins, 21, 22, 24
Baby Kale Salad with Pine Nuts and Blueberries, 84
bacteria, in digestive system, 6, 21
baked foods vs. fried/grilled foods, 17
baking basics
  about, 27
  grinding gluten-free flours, 33
  key ingredients, 31–33
  tips, 27–31
baking mixes, 28
baking pans, 29
baking powder, 28
Banana Bread, 56
barley, 20
Bars, Crispy Rice, 145
Bars, Puffy, 144
Basic Three-Layer White Cake, 124–125
Basic Two-Layer White Cake, 122–123
basmati rice, 23
batters, safety and, 28
bean flours, as gluten-free, 11
beans, 20. *See also* specific types of
Bhutan, red rice from, 24
Bisque, Creamy Carrot, with Exotic Spices, 93
Bisque, Quick Broccoli, 92
Black Bean Tostadas, 102–103
black forbidden rice, 24
Blank-Slate Quick Bread, 52–53
blend(s)
  All-Purpose Herb, 46
  Creole Spice, 43
  Ethiopian Spice Mix, 48
  Five-Alarm Chili Powder, 45

Garam Masala, 42
Italian Seasoning, 47
Kick-it-Up Spice, 44
Sweet-and-Hot Mix, 49
Blendtec kitchen mill/ blender, 33
bloating, 2
blood tests, for celiac disease, 3
Blueberries, Baby Kale Salad with Pine Nuts and, 84
Blueberry Streusel Coffee Cake, 130–131
bone/joint pain, 2
bowel disease, 2
Bragg Liquid Aminos, 20
breadings/coatings on foods, 16
bread(s)
  Banana, 56
  Blank-Slate Quick, 52–53
  Chapatis, Gluten-Free, 58–59
  Cornbread Squares, 60
  Crêpes, Chickpea, 61
  injera, 24
  muffins
    Chocolate, 53
    Cinnamon-Raisin, 53
    Crunchy Seed or Nut, 53
    Dilly, 53
    Dried Fruit, 53
    Lemon-Poppy Seed, 53
    Magical One-Bowl, 52
    Maple Corn, 53
    Marmalade, 53
    Onion-Herb, 53
    Orange, 53
    Quinoa-Corn, 53
  Pancakes, Silver Dollar, 62
  Pumpkin Spice, 54–55
  Scones, Vanilla-Currant, 57
  Sunny Seed, 51
breakfast recipes

ABOUT THE AUTHOR

Jo Stepaniak is the author and coauthor of more than two dozen books on vegan cuisine, health, and compassionate living. She has dealt with multiple food sensitivities and understands firsthand the challenges of living with dietary restrictions.

Book Publishing Co.

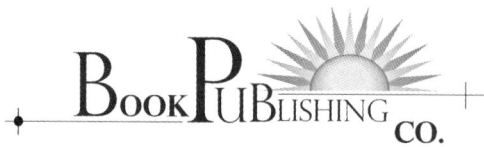

books that educate, inspire, and empower

To find your favorite books on plant-based cooking and nutrition,
living foods lifestyle, and healthy living,
visit BookPubCo.com

Sign up for our free online Healthy Living Newsletter to get delicious recipes and health tips.

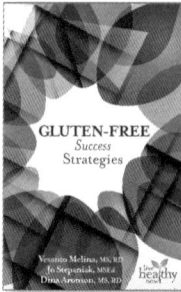

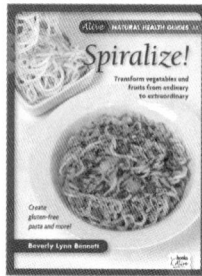

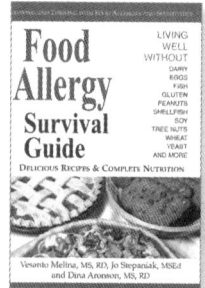

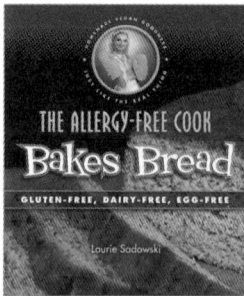

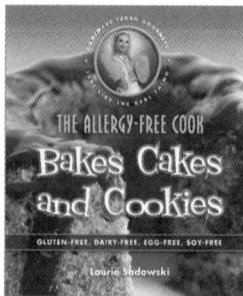

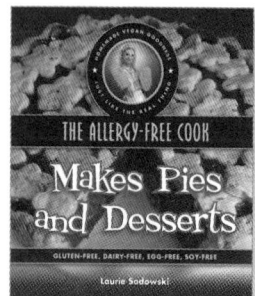